Sawdust and Turnip Greens

A Compilation of Columns Published In the Brentwood Homepage

Bill Fleet

PUBLISHED BY WESTVIEW, INC.
KINGSTON SPRINGS, TENNESSEE

Published by Westview, Inc.
P.O. Box 605
Kingston Springs, TN 37082
www.publishedbywestview.com

ISBN 978-1-62880-009-8

First edition, September 2013

The author gratefully acknowledges permission from Susan Leathers to reprint these articles, which were first printed in the *Brentwood Journal.*

Printed in the United States of America on acid free paper.

To S.R. Lee (Sally)
Scholar, Teacher, Poet, Friend

Introduction

One of the saddest comments I heard at my thirtieth medical-school reunion was by the wife of one of my old classmates. She said, "Bob doesn't do anything but sit on the couch and watch soap operas all day." Several times in the years before I retired, thoughts ran through my mind about what I would do when I no longer worked at a steady job. Would I be terminally bored like my classmate, or would I stay busy? Busy won out. My days are full. Though it seems I seldom get anything done, just being busy is enough.

Before I retired, I spent free time in my woodworking shop in winter, and in my vegetable garden and Carolyn's flowerbed in summer. I have persisted in both hobbies, though I have cut back on the volume of work as I approached eighty.

Three years ago I learned of a new e-paper service covering my hometown. I asked the editor for a job as a feature columnist. The editor said, "Send me two pieces and we will decide." I did that, and she asked me to do a weekly column. Later, she asked me the name of my column-to-be and I answered with some longish title. She replied, "Give me something shorter." "Sawdust and Turnip Greens" popped into my head. At least it reflected two of my three hobbies.

I had free rein of subject and the paper had free use of my services. This book is a compilation of some of those columns. Almost all the articles are as true as I can remember the truth. A few are mostly true. A rare piece is pure fabrication, and I have identified those stories that are mostly fiction. Most of those are located in the section on childhood memories.

I am grateful to Susan Leathers, editor of the *Brentwood Journal* for allowing me to reprint these columns from the publication.

Bill Fleet

Chapter One, Pediatrics

My pediatric experience spans forty years if one includes the time spent in clinical and research training and the nine years of research and teaching as a full-time member of the pediatric faculty at Vanderbilt. I ended my career as a general pediatrician practitioner. Teaching and research remained a small but vital part of those twenty-five years. Most of the stories in this chapter are memories from those last twenty-five years.

Adventures in the Delivery Room and Beyond

As a pediatrician, people often confused me with an obstetrician. Over and over I heard, "It must be so satisfying to deliver babies." I never wanted to deliver babies; I never wanted to do surgery. I loved the babies. Even though I did not like obstetrics, I spent a lot of time in delivery rooms. Since about ten percent of babies are born with problems, I was in a delivery room about once a week.

Multiple births drew me to delivery rooms with regularity. Twin births usually presented few difficulties. I could stabilize one twin while a nurse from the newborn nursery dealt with the other. Of course, if they were born sick, I had to deal with both, simultaneously, with help from a nursery nurse or two.

One New Year's Day, my major referring obstetrician called. "I'm going to deliver triplets this afternoon. You probably should be here."

Probably? Triplets were certain to require resuscitation and major medical support. They were almost guaranteed to be very small and in severe distress. "Is the mother too near delivery to transfer to Vandy?" I asked.

He replied, "I've never delivered triplets and I want to deliver them here."

He could not be dissuaded. The mother delivered three boys, all weighing five pounds or so, all pink, all vigorous, all squirming, all crying. Two years later, the triplets had a new brother. I could always tell when they were in my office: every movable object in their exam room had been moved to the hall.

"Natural childbirth" became high fashion during my working life. Lamaze was on everyone's lips. Giving a mother so much as Tylenol was frowned upon. Epidurals were for wimps.

One night, I was called to attend the delivery of a baby who was thought likely to need special care after delivery. I arrived shortly before the birth, and the poor mother was exhausted from her lengthy labor. Finally, she asked for an epidural and pain medication. Her husband bent down and said, "Oh, no. You don't need anything. The baby will be here soon." She looked up at him, made a fist, and BAM! Socked him right in the mouth. I thought her response was quite appropriate.

Toward the end of my private practice career, most outlying hospitals had acquired some type of neonatology coverage. Unfortunately, one of my hospitals resisted this innovation.

I attended a delivery there when resuscitation might be needed. Fortunately, it wasn't. I suctioned the baby's nose and mouth, dried her off, wrapped her in warm blankets, and, after she became acquainted with her parents, I carried her in my arms across the hall to the nursery. As usual, I ran a gauntlet of anxious family and friends. As I fought my way through the throng, someone asked, "Are you the neonatologist?" Of course, the hospital had not a single neonatologist.

I replied, "You bet—the best one in this hospital."

After a sick baby had been resuscitated and stabilized in the delivery room, further evaluation and therapy was usually required, often in the neonatal intensive care unit at Vanderbilt. Late one night, after I had stabilized a sick newborn, I called Angel 1, the Vandy transport team. Since it takes more than an hour for the team to arrive in their specially appointed ambulance, I pulled off my shoes and socks and crawled into a bed in a labor room across the hall for a short nap. (I was still in my scrub suit that I had worn in the delivery room and could be back in the nursery immediately if the baby developed problems.) When the Vandy team arrived, I padded across the hall into the nursery without benefit of either shoes or socks, and discussed the baby with the female neonatologist, who happened to also be a good friend of mine.

The next week, on my afternoon off, I was playing tennis when paged. I hurried off to the same hospital for "fetal distress." This baby was, indeed, in distress and needed me. He was limp, blue, and not breathing, but his heart rate was normal—at least one good sign. I intubated him, attached a resuscitation bag to the endotracheal tube, and began to ventilate him. Once he became pink and regained some muscle tone, I carried him to the nursery, where I inserted a catheter into one of his umbilical arteries to monitor his metabolic recovery. (Catheterizing a newborn baby's umbilical artery is slightly more difficult than giving an enema to an earthworm.)

After that, I called for Angel 1. When they came, the same female neonatologist was on the team. I described what I had done and what the current data showed, and stood in the nursery dressed in my tennis shorts covered by one of those dreadful, backless hospital gowns.

She patiently listened to my spiel, accepted copies of all the data we had generated so far, and huffed, in her best pseudo-insulted voice, "Last week, I came here and you had no shoes. Today, you have no pants. I'm not coming here ever again!"

Babies

I spent forty years as a pediatrician. I didn't deliver babies. I took care of babies' medical needs. My field was children of all ages, from birth to young adulthood. People often exclaimed, "Oh, you are a baby doctor!"

I replied, "No. I'm fully grown."

People often presented their newly born grandchildren to me stating, "Don't you think he's (she's) the prettiest baby you have ever seen?" As a pediatrician, I saw quite a few newborn babies. To be truthful, they mostly looked very similar to each other. They are red-faced, with eyes closed, arms and legs flexed, hands making tiny fists, and they are often crying. These are the normal ones.

I heard, "Doesn't he look just like his mama (daddy, grandparent, Aunt Susie, etc.)?" And of course, he does, but so do most of the babies in the nursery, if you look closely. They all have two eyes, two hands and feet, and a single nose and chin. Often the nose is crooked, pushed to one side like the loser in a boxing match, but family members can always dredge up a resemblance to some relative or other.

Most newborns resemble each other closely. Only a few stand out. There are a few babies that indeed are pretty—even beautiful—but those are few. Most fall into the category of "generic baby."

There are also a very few who are ugly. No other way to describe them except ugly. The poor things cannot help it. They have no pleasing facial features, are just redder and crying harder and with a more severely misshapen nose than most babies. Occasionally, they have linear bruises on their faces from the pressure of forceps. The most reassuring feature they have is that their looks will always change with time.

When the grandparent of one of those babies asks, "Don't you think he's beautiful?" I am hard put to agree. There is a limit to how much I can suspend reality. Early in my practice, I didn't know just what to reply. Usually I mumbled something that satisfied neither the grandparent nor me. Finally, I came upon a reply that I could live with. When faced with one of those lovable but less-than-attractive babies, I would reply, "That's a real baby."

Swaddling Cloths

"You will find a child wrapped in bands of cloth…" Luke 2:12 (NRSV). How many times have you read or heard this quoted, either as "swaddling cloths" or "swaddling clothes"? They are an integral part of the Christmas story. You can't have a Christmas story without swaddling cloths. But have you ever seen any?

I hadn't until over thirty years ago, when I was on the faculty of Vanderbilt medical school and was asked to join a team of physicians to evaluate the medical needs of children in Algiers. I jumped at the chance to visit a country few Americans ever see—and with all expenses paid.

I landed at the airport in Algiers midmorning, expecting a representative of my group to meet me. None was to be seen. I was on my own in a foreign country, a country hostile to the United States where English was not a second language. After several minutes of gesturing and shouting, I made a cabby aware of my destination, the Walaia, the governor's offices. A cab deposited me in downtown Algiers far from the governor's office.

I wandered through narrow streets filled with cars, trucks, donkey carts, and buses. Robed men cruised the sidewalks and veiled women walked with heads bowed close to buildings. I expected to see Humphrey Bogart or Ingrid Bergman at any moment. Finally, I saw a small sign saying, "Walaia." I had found my goal—the Walaia.

I entered through a plain door into a large, shabby lobby filled with people standing in long lines before a room-wide counter. Bored clerks stood behind the counter stamping one form after another.

Suddenly, a strong hand grabbed my elbow in a vise-like grip. I was quickly propelled into a small room and questioned for over an hour about my intentions in the country. After I had convinced the intelligence officer of my legitimate reasons for being in his country, he directed me to my hotel, where I finally met the rest of my group. Our liaison officer explained that I had entered the public area of the complex and not the diplomatic area. I had been glaringly out of place. I was lucky not to have been jailed.

Since I was the lone pediatrician in our delegation, I concentrated on children's hospitals and clinics. Almost every infant was wrapped in swaddling cloths consisting of tight bindings around the trunk, from shoulders to ankles, including the arms. Because of less-than-perfect hygiene, many babies had diaper rash from chin to ankles.

Several years later, during my teaching rounds at Vanderbilt Children's Hospital, I was shown an infant with a severe, angry, red eruption involving his entire trunk from shoulders to ankles. Nobody had any idea of what strange malady this infant suffered. Even dermatologists were stumped. The baby was scheduled for a skin biopsy that day.

I looked the baby over and asked one question: "Is this baby a Kurdish refugee?"

"Yes."

"I believe you should cancel the biopsy. This child has diaper rash."

And so the baby did.

All Part of the Job

Every profession requires special skills. The medical field is broad, and necessary skills depend upon the medical field the physician enters. Surgeons require fine motor skills of varying types and all surgeons require unshakable self-confidence. An open chest or abdomen or beating heart are not places for the faint of heart (pun intended).

Internists need patience to listen to varying—and sometimes obscure—symptoms and need the intellectual skills to assemble seemingly unrelated findings into an integrated whole.

And then there are pediatricians—among whom I toiled for forty years. Everyone decries the fact that my little patients cannot tell me their symptoms. Do not worry. We substitute observation for oral complaints. We know a one-year-old lying quietly in her mother's lap, unresisting to gentle examination and uninterested in her surroundings, is likely to be quite ill. The pink, screaming, kicking fighter may well be quite healthy.

We pediatricians develop subtle ways of examining our patients as gently as we can. Much of the exam can be done with the infant lying in his mother's lap.

There are special motor skills pediatricians need. Collecting a blood sample from most adults is simple and easily done. Finding a vein in a chubby, screaming, fighting eighteen-month-old is another matter altogether. I realized early in my career that the nurse holding the baby is usually more important to successful procedures than the person on the business end of the needle.

There is one manual skill I developed that I think might have been unique. I could open a locked car door without a key almost as easily as the average car thief. About once or twice a year, usually on a hot summer day, a frantic mother came into our office crying, asking for help. She had locked her infant in her car.

Almost always the story went like this: The mother and infant had finished seeing their pediatrician, and the dutiful mother unlocked the car, laid her purse on the front seat, and proceeded to strap the baby into the car seat. Then she closed the car door with her purse and key lying on the seat, and the door locked automatically. She always beat a hasty retreat into our office for help.

A call to a locksmith would produce one in a half-hour or so, but an infant in a closed car on a hot day can be in trouble in a short time. I kept a straightened coat hanger in a closet and learned to unlock car doors with a minimum of effort.

Toward the end of my practice, car door locks became impossible to open with a coat hanger. Luckily, I met the challenge. My sister was the town clerk in my small hometown. One of her duties was to supervise the town's three police officers. She kept a slim metal tool designed for defeating car door locks. When the city bought new up-to-date tools, she gave me the old ones. I was quite successful using them.

I never needed that tool more than a few times a year, but it resulted in a rescued baby and a grateful mother. The service was free. Medical insurance refused to pay. They don't have a code number for breaking into cars.

Fat Children

Michelle Obama, you go girl! You started a campaign against childhood obesity today. Finally, the problem of fat children has reached national attention.

What welcomed news! I fought fat for over twenty-five years of my pediatric practice with spectacular lack of success. And there were plenty of battles to fight. It is estimated that about one-third of American children today are overweight, and about half of them are obese. We know our population is growing fatter and fatter, and children are part of the problem.

The causes of obesity are obvious. If we put more calories into our bodies than we burn in physical activity, the excess calories will be converted to fat. If we eat too much and exercise too little, we make fat. Air conditioning and television keep children indoors, on the couch, and eating—and often high calorie fatty or sugary foods. My prejudice against air conditioning is probably fostered by my non-air conditioned childhood. I remember sweating a lot, but don't remember being hot. But of course I can't do without my air conditioning now that I am in my senior years.

Also, overweight parents tend to have overweight children. I think part of the cause is a genetic tendency for overweight persons to metabolize foods more efficiently than their thinner contemporaries—but not all. Overweight people often underestimate their caloric intake.

Here is a true-life example. I saw a five-year-old boy for his preschool exam one day. He weighed about sixty-five pounds when he should have weighed about forty-five. I pointed this fact out to his chubby mother.

She replied, "I just don't understand. He hardly eats anything."

I asked, "What did he eat for breakfast this morning?"

"He had sausage and biscuits and gravy. He loves that and eats it almost every morning."

"How about lunch?"

"He had a McDonald's cheeseburger and fries and a milkshake."

"What was for supper last night?"

"Oh, we had pizza."

"How many slices did he have?"

"He ate the whole thing… but it was only a small one."

The Joys of Pediatrics

Infants and children exhibit ever-changing characteristics. They change physically, but they also change their behavior patterns. They go from nonresponsive newborns to smiling six-month-olds to crying, uncooperative challenges from ages one to about three. By three, I could jolly them along and receive a modicum of cooperation.

But by four years, they are delights. I loved to see four-year-olds. Here are a few stories from my four year-old patients.

Jason got up listless, refused breakfast, and complained of a stomachache. He had no fever or other symptoms. His mother allowed him to stay home. By midmorning, he was playing outside, even climbing trees. His mother dressed him, and as they drove to daycare he turned to her and asked, "Would an earache have been better?"

My third-year student asked another four-year-old, "Let me see if I can hear Barney in your heart."

She replied, "Oh no, I have Jesus in my heart. I have Barney in my panties."

Part of my routine in well-child visits was to obtain a rough idea of the child's developmental progress. Four-year-olds are supposed to be able to identify colors, so I usually asked about them.

One little girl replied, "Of course I know my colors. Red and yellow and blue are primary colors, purple and orange are secondary colors, and gray is a neutral color."

I told her mother, “All I was after was a yes or no, not a lecture.” I had forgotten her mother was an artist.

I asked another four-year-old boy once, “What makes a sailboat go?”

He said, “I’m not exactly sure, but I think the wind pressure is higher on one side of the sail and lower on the other, and that makes the sail push the boat.”

I expected “wind” or “sails” and not another lecture.

I had a few patients who were difficult to deal with, but most were a delight. As a pediatrician for forty years, I was puzzled sometimes, I was frustrated sometimes, but I was bored, never.

The Job Interview

We needed help. The three of us in our pediatric practice had become so busy that a fourth doctor was our only solution for surviving the upcoming winter's crush of sick children.

We talked with several Vanderbilt faculty members, and it seemed that Rich was the best candidate from their excellent pediatric training program.

Rich spent an afternoon with us at our office during his second visit. He seemed interested. He looked good to us. We decided to offer him a job.

Rich and I met for a typical pediatric power lunch—sandwiches and sodas in our conference room. After we had finished lunch, I began to lay out our offer. Partway through my spiel my nurse interrupted the meeting saying, "Dr. Fleet, you have a new patient in the treatment room and you need to see her right now." My nurse had been with me for almost twenty years and knew her pediatrics. When she said "now," it was time for me to move, and move quickly.

Rich and I hurried across the hall into the treatment room to encounter a pale, blue, limp two-week-old baby gasping for air. She was dying in her mother's arms.

My nurse had already begun oxygen. Tools for tracheal intubation and a proper size oxygen bag and mask lay on the treatment table beside needles for IVs. IV fluids hung beside the table ready to be connected.

I asked a few questions of the mother, made a few comforting noises, and made a quick examination.

Everything pointed toward a severe cardiac problem that was dependent on an open ductus arterosus (a large artery essential during prenatal life that closes at around two weeks when it is no longer needed). The baby had been thrown into severe heart failure by the closure of the ductus. Reopening the ductus with a medication would buy time for surgeons to repair the heart defect. This medication is not available in outpatient settings. The baby would have to go to Vanderbilt with all possible speed. But first, the baby had to live to get there.

We quickly prepared to place a tube in the infant's windpipe. I deferred to Rich. His skill at this rather difficult procedure was honed sharper than ours, since he was actively training in a hospital setting.

Rich tried twice without success. One of my associates slipped the tube into the windpipe as quickly and skillfully as if she were giving a bottle to hungry baby.

While the intubation was proceeding, my other associate inserted a needle into a vein and attached the IV fluids. I stood beside the table directing the activities—a mundane but very important role in a resuscitation. I was thinking. Everyone else was doing.

An ambulance arrived as we finished our work. I called Vanderbilt as everyone left, warned them of the critically ill infant on her way, and suggested they have available a vial of the drug to open the ductus ready when she arrived.

The office crisis was over. Everyone took a deep breath, and weak smiles flitted across several faces. Seldom are we privileged to save a life so decisively, and our personnel had met the challenge—and passed—when it counted.

Rich and I strolled back into the conference room. We sat down, I exhaled forcefully and said, "Rich, we seldom examine our candidates so severely but you seemed to be a special case."

❦

Note to the reader: The Vanderbilt Pediatric Emergency physicians met the baby at the door and started the drug I had suggested, and within a few minutes, the baby began to kick and squirm, to breathe easily, and to try to cry in spite of the tube in her windpipe. Surgery that day partially corrected the baby's heart defect. Unfortunately, she died about a month later of complications of a second surgery.

We offered Rich the job. He took it.

Ingestions

Children eat the craziest things, and often refuse what is good—giving some credence to the adage that children are merely small adults.

During my first summer in practice, I received a call one morning. "My baby has just eaten some grass killer. What should I do?"

Recalling a recent experience with a fatal case of grass killer ingestion, I almost shouted, "Bring him in as quickly as you can; be sure to bring in the original container to identify the poison!" After what seemed a long wait, my patient arrived. He seemed normal to my quick exam.

"Where is the grass killer container?" I demanded.

"It's out in the truck," his mother explained.

"Well, bring it right in!"

"But it's a thirty-gallon drum."

The poison was only granular calcium chlorate, a salt-like chemical that can kill grass in addition to its other uses. Taken in small amounts, it is harmless to humans. This was the first of many ingestion calls I received in my years of practice.

Another unusual dietary indiscretion also occurred early in my career. One evening about suppertime, I received a call. "My two-year old just ate a tablespoonful of instant coffee powder. What should I do?"

I knew the mother well, and also knew that the amount of coffee ingested would, at worst, only cause sleeplessness. I advised, "Give him some cream and sugar and he should be okay."

His mother called in a few hours to give a progress report, as I had requested. "He seems okay, but I gave him some water after I talked with you, and he perked."

We were taught to avoid leading questions when taking a medical history. Rather than asking, "Does your abdomen hurt under your ribs?" we were taught to ask, "Where do you hurt?" However, when confronted with a child suspected of ingesting a prescription or an illicit drug, I soon learned to make my questions more direct, like the kind one hears on police television shows. I frequently used the following two cases to illustrate this technique to students and residents.

Late one afternoon, I received a call from a nearby hospital emergency department. "We have a child here in coma and need your help right away," a nurse said in a worried voice.

I rushed to the hospital and found a three-year-old boy who was unconscious. He was pink and breathing easily, his blood pressure was normal, and he bore no signs of trauma. He roused somewhat and protested when disturbed, but soon lapsed back into his unconscious state when left alone. I soon realized the child was not sick but only deeply sedated.

I asked his parents, "Is there any way he could have taken any medications at home?"

"Oh, no. We don't have any medicines in the house."

"Don't you have aspirin or Tylenol or Advil?"

"Oh, sure. We have those things."

"Any sleeping pills?"

"No."

"Any nerve pills?"

"No."

"Was there anyone else in the house today?"

"His great aunt stayed with him for me this afternoon."

"Does she take any pills?"

"I think she does, but she would never leave them where my baby could get them."

"Would you call her and ask her if there was any way one of her pills could have gotten into your son's hands?" I handed his mother a telephone and stood by while she called.

"She said she took a nerve pill while at our house."

"Ask her if she might have dropped one."

"She said she thought she might have, but she couldn't find it on the floor."

I knew who found it.

Another evening I was called to the same emergency department to see an unconscious two-year-old. Again, a careful exam revealed no serious findings except that the child was unconscious and appeared sedated. I began my questions to the parents. "Is there any way he could have taken any medicines?"

"No."

"Do you have any medicines in the house?"

"No."

"Do you take nerve pills or sleeping pills?"

"No."

"Have you ever taken nerve pills or sleeping pills?"

"Yes, but not for several months."

"Did you have any pills left over?"
"Yes, but I threw them away."
"When did you throw them away?"
"Last week."
"Where did you throw them?"
"In the trash can."
"Did you empty the trash can?"
"Not yet."

Adolescent Medicine

Teenagers don't fit anywhere. They despise sitting in pediatricians' waiting rooms filled with babies and young children, and are uncomfortable in internists' waiting rooms filled with people with canes and walkers and Medicare. Bookcases in pediatrician's offices are usually filled with books and magazines on childcare and behavior with a sprinkling of children's books. Internists' offices are usually limited to magazines of more mature interest such as investments, retirement, and news.

Televisions play in both offices, but programs usually provide cartoons or game shows. (I wish there were places in internists' and surgeons' waiting rooms that are TV-free, but I have yet to find one.)

At the time I was in school and in postgraduate training, few medical schools and pediatric training programs made a significant effort to deal with adolescents as a group deserving special attention and expertise. Many schools and training programs shunted children to internists after their twelfth birthday. However, by the time I had set up my practice, adolescent medicine had emerged as a valid and useful area of practice. My lack of skill with adolescents prompted me to attend conferences, lectures, and reading on the subject, and as time passed, my younger associates added to my understanding of the unique and changing physical and emotional needs of this age group.

My first office was typical of pediatric offices of the day—no place for adolescents. When we planned our new office to accommodate three or four physicians, we designed an area to meet the needs of this unique population.

We had three rooms equipped with exam tables suitable for adults and adaptable for gynecological exams. There was a separate waiting room for adolescents, equipped with TV, stereo, and magazines of interest to teens. There were brochures on the dangers of sexually-transmitted diseases and the dangers of smoking, drinking, and the use of cellphones while driving. Whether these tracts were helpful I do not know, but they were more suitable for this age than nursery rhymes.

I called this area of our office our "geriatric section."

Commuting

There was an article published recently about the horrendous traffic jam and gridlock outside of Beijing, China. Those poor commuters were stuck in a ten-day, sixty- mile traffic jam triggered by road repairs. And I thought I had it tough during my decades commuting twenty-five miles through Nashville from Brentwood to Goodlettsville!

I still pity the poor commuters living north and east of Nashville. Hardly a day goes by without a report of a traffic-slowing crash on I-65 north or I-40 east of town. Sometimes there is more than one accident and sometimes there are accidents on both commuter arteries simultaneously—but nothing approaching the situation in Beijing. Drivers slept on the pavement or played cards beside their vehicles. Authorities have been only partially successful in alleviating future similar occurrences.

Over the twenty-five years of commuting, I had only a single significant accident myself.

Late one February afternoon, I entered south on the interstate at Goodlettsville, and just as I reached traffic speed, a blue blur flashed across my vision. It was followed by a deafening crash, and a huge projectile smashed my windshield. I awoke to a man knocking on my window asking, "Are you all right?"

I assured him I was fine and I replaced my glasses that had flown off because of the sudden deceleration. As I stepped out, I remembered I hadn't turned off my headlights, and I didn't want to run my battery down.

Then I realized I had no headlights and no battery to run down. The entire front of my car had disintegrated. A car engine lay partway through the windshield on my passenger side.

As I slowly regained my senses, I saw a blue sedan lying partly under an upset semi-trailer in the right southbound lane, a boat lying off its trailer in the median, a pickup stalled across both northbound lanes, and a car stopped on the shoulder of the interstate heading north. In all, there were five vehicles and a boat blocking the interstate in both directions.

It took several highway patrolmen about an hour to investigate the accident and to supervise clearing the interstate. According to their report, the blue sedan was pulling the boat north at high rate of speed and ran into the pickup, which was slowed by exiting traffic. The sedan driver lost control, veered into the median, lost his trailer, and entered the southbound lanes where I hit him broadside at sixty miles per hour. The collision knocked the sedan under the semi-trailer which, before it capsized, knocked the sedan's engine completely out. The engine flew into my windshield, and the oil filter flew back across the median and through the driver's side window, spewing oil over the interior of the northbound car.

I walked away with just a bruised chest from the impact of the seatbelt. The only significant injury in the entire melee was the sedan driver's fractured ankle. My bank account didn't fare too well, though. My car was totaled. If I had known the sedan driver had only the minimum liability insurance, he might have had a head injury as well.

I missed my tennis date that night, but I did go to work the next day.

Give thanks for seatbelts.

Adventures while Making Hospital Rounds

The Gravel Truck Wreck

One fall morning I stopped as the second car behind a traffic light. While I waited impatiently, I noticed a loaded articulated sixteen-wheel gravel truck careening down the side street at a high rate of speed. As the truck attempted to make a right turn onto our street, it tipped over. The gravel-filled trailer landed on the car in front of me, smashing it down like someone stepping on a drink can. The truck ended up on its side next to my car, leaking fuel. I jumped out of my car and heard the truck driver complaining of pain in his shoulder and asking for help. I yelled to him to get himself out. (If he were alert and moving both arms and legs, he couldn't be too severely injured.) I ran to the smashed car in front of me expecting to find a dead or severely injured driver.

The car was flattened down to the level of the hood, and in it, a woman lay on her side across the front seat. As soon as I opened what was left of the passenger door, she looked up at me and complained about pain in her legs. I immediately thought, "If she can complain, she is alert, and at least does not have a significant brain injury." When she could move her feet and toes at my request, I knew she probably did not have a significant spinal cord injury, either. She could not slide out of the car, however, because the steering wheel had been crushed down onto her thighs, pinning her to the front seat.

Just as I arrived at the conclusion that she was not seriously injured, a man holding a smoldering cigarette came up behind me to help. I could smell and see gasoline on the street and in the gutter. I screamed, "Get away from the street and put that cigarette out!" (What a tragedy if a fire should start while the woman was trapped in the car!) After he had safely extinguished his cigarette, I assigned him to be fire prevention officer.

Soon a thoracic surgeon friend of mine arrived. He had stopped at the scene, knowing there might be little any layman could do in accidents like this. He agreed that the pinned driver seemed not to be severely injured. I stayed at her side, trying to keep her from becoming too upset, when suddenly, a hand grabbed my shoulder and thrust me aside. A voice behind me shouted, "Get out of the way! I'm a nurse's aide!"

I turned and said, "Thank you for coming. Take over." I turned the patient over to her and backed away, grateful for relief.

I waited until the extraction unit arrived to pry the woman out. She walked to the waiting ambulance!

The Motorcycle Wreck

I have never been able to pass a highway accident without stopping. Every time, I felt almost helpless. The lack of equipment and supplies prevented me from doing more than primitive Boy-Scout-type first aid. Even so, I always stopped. I have stopped at several car-motorcycle confrontations, and the car always won.

One day while on my way to make hospital rounds, I encountered such an accident. As I sat at a traffic light on the main highway to Hendersonville, I saw a motorcycle. Just as he approached the red light, I looked to my left, and, to my horror, saw a car enter the intersection on a collision course with the motorcycle. The motorcycle ran head-on into the car. The rider made a complete flip over the car and landed face-first onto the street beside me.

I began to assess the damage. The motorcycle rider lay in the street moaning and bleeding from his mouth. His helmet visor was cracked and askew on his head. I feared a significant upper spinal cord injury and forbade anyone to move him until the ambulance and emergency medical personnel arrived. After he was on his way to the hospital, I left the scene, made my hospital rounds, and then detoured through the emergency area to check on the motorcyclist. I found him sitting on a stretcher, with his only injury a lacerated tongue.

Keep Your Seatbelts On!

One Christmas Eve morning, I received an emergency page as I made hospital rounds before going to my office. Two of my patients and their mother were in the emergency department at Hendersonville Hospital following an automobile accident. I was asked to go there as soon as possible. I found a mother with a broken leg; her two-year-old daughter was crying because of pain from bruises inflicted by her seatbelt straps. The child was otherwise unhurt. The four-year-old boy was dead from a broken neck. He hated his seatbelt and was allowed to stand on the floor resting his chin on the dashboard, looking out as his mother drove. His only visible injury was a small bruise on his chin. The blow had broken his neck. There was no way I could break the news to his mother that would minimize her pain.

Mamas, make your children grow up wearing seatbelts!

The Good Samaritan?

West Side Hospital (now part of the Centennial Hospital complex) had a doctors' lounge with a small buffet that served excellent free breakfasts and lunches to the doctors on the hospital staff. I developed the habit of arising early and simply drinking a cup of coffee on the way to Vanderbilt, Baptist, and West Side hospitals. After rounds, I then dropped in to the West Side doctors' lounge for breakfast. A middle-aged lady tended the breakfast buffet, cleaned the tables, and greeted each new arrival. She had developed an easy, casual friendship with the regular breakfast clientele.

One morning I noticed our attendant leaning against the refrigerator with tears streaming down her cheeks. I recalled the subject of our last Sunday School lesson about making the first move toward people who were in pain, and hesitantly walked over to her.

"Have you received some bad news? Is there anything I can do to help?" I asked.

She turned, blotted her eyes and replied, "No. I was cutting grapefruit and got some of the juice in my eyes."

She always served me choice items from the breakfast buffet from that day on.

If the Disease Fits…

Some several years ago when I was still gainfully employed and contributing to the Gross Domestic Product a bit, I came upon an unusual situation. It happened something like this.

My son, Bill, and his wife and boys left their geriatric Labrador named Susie with us while out of town on vacation. Bill told us that Susie had seemed rather lethargic for a few days, and if her symptoms persisted, based on previous illness and behaviors, they thought she had a urinary tract infection.

Susie continued to be lethargic, and underwent a two-day self-imposed fast. I started her on some amoxicillin antibiotic, chosen because it should be effective and I had a good supply of samples in my office. After two days of treatment, she returned to her previous levels of activity and appetite. I stopped her meds after a week. I assumed she was cured even though she took child medicine rather than dog medicine.

A few days later, I saw one of my favorite families. There were four healthy girls with an attractive, lively mother whose every sentence seemed to be accompanied by laughter. They always brightened my day with each visit. The father was a veterinarian with a busy practice in a nearby town.

That Monday morning, I saw the youngest daughter. She was about seven years old, and had a fever and a sore throat for three days over a winter weekend. Her mother said, "Leslie complained of a sore throat Friday night and developed a fever Saturday. Her father did a strep test on her Saturday, and it showed strep. He started her on some of his veterinary amoxicillin Saturday. She seems better today, but I brought her in anyway."

I peered at her reddened throat and thought, "Leslie, Susie. People meds for a dog. Dog meds for people." Something seemed wrong somehow, but both were well in only a few days.

Angel Parents

The story by Mrs. Larisa Helsinki in last week's Brentwood Homepage about her daughter's positive experience with the staff of the Children's Hospital reminded me of some of my experiences with patients during my pediatric practice. The following describes some of my angel parents. Lack of room prevents me from describing them all.

Early in my practice, I saw a newly-born infant in one of the local hospitals. He had all the typical findings of Down syndrome. After my exam, I made my way to the mother's room reluctantly. I sat down and told the young couple of their baby's condition and his prognosis. They accepted my diagnosis with aplomb. During our conversation I began to wonder if they really understood the implications of the diagnosis. Many people hear but don't comprehend bad news when it is first presented.

Later, during well-child visits, I discussed the possibilities of their future children having the same syndrome. Younger parents with one Down baby are more likely than the general population to have another Down baby. Although they were aware of accurate prenatal diagnosis of Down syndrome, the family declined. They said, "There's no need to have the test. We will love all our babies just the way we love their brother." The family had three more children. All were well.

Those parents were instrumental in developing the Middle Tennessee Down Association, a parent support group. There was no parent support group available previously. Their son graduated from high school after passing the statewide required exams.

Mrs. R. led an altogether usual life—for a time. She was married to a lineman employed by the Nashville Electric Service. She had a daughter and was pregnant with twins when her husband touched the wrong wire and suffered a near-fatal accident. He was left with significant mobility difficulties and frequent seizures.

One twin developed diabetes when she was about two years old. She required strict dietary control, frequent finger sticks to measure blood sugar levels, and at least two injections of insulin per day. Since there was no parental support group in Middle Tennessee, Mrs. R. started the Middle Tennessee Juvenile Diabetes Association. Under her guidance, the group developed a newsletter and organized summer camps for diabetic children.

Mrs. R. designed and sewed a stuffed animal, a "Sugar Bug", for her daughter to "inject" when she received her own insulin. It is now available nationwide.

The B. family already had two healthy children when their son was born. He was born with a rare syndrome that resulted in severe feeding difficulties, chronic severe pulmonary problems, and a marked developmental delay. By the extraordinary efforts of his parents, he lived to age twenty-seven when the average life span was thirteen. His parents became a major voice in the Associations of

Retarded Citizens (state and national), and are still active in those organizations.

These are only three families. I could describe many.

About ten percent of people are saints, ten percent are a pain in the neck, and the rest of us are somewhere in between. I have been blessed and humbled to have known so many in that first group.

Victory

There is no victory without a winner. But not all winners are victors in a game or contest. Some winners have conquered adversity within themselves. I know of such a winner.

One busy morning at my office, my nurse handed me a chart and said, "Your next patient is new. He's a two-week-old foster child. His foster mother is with him. She's blind."

I said, "Blind? A foster mother? How does she manage? What does Human Services mean by using a blind foster mother? There's no way a blind mother can take care of a newborn baby."

I entered Room Ten and introduced myself to Mrs. G. She reached out and shook my hand. After examining the information supplied by Human Services, I asked Mrs. G. to undress the baby. She removed all the baby's clothes skillfully and laid each item on the end of the exam table.

After my exam, we discussed baby care and schedules for well-baby visits. She assured me she could manage the baby and that transportation to the office would not be a problem.

I said, "You can dress him now." I watched closely as she dressed him, including putting his little socks on his feet. She picked up each item of clothing from the pile and put it on him without fumbling once.

I thought, "There's no way this woman is blind. No blind person can dress a baby like that."

As she turned to leave she ran full force into the wall next to the exam room door. I thought, "I guess she is blind after all."

She managed the baby without a problem, and over the next years cared for five others, sometimes more than one at a time. Once she even became upset when she failed to diagnose a case of diaper rash in one of her babies. Mrs. G. was a winner. I kept score.

Surprises

My life as a pediatrician was seldom dull. Even routine well-baby visits sometimes contained surprises.

Early in my practice career, I met the parents of a new baby in the hospital. Both husband and wife accompanied their baby to her first checkup at age two weeks. The baby was progressing well and the few problems they had were minor.

Both parents were dressed casually in faded, frayed jeans. The mother had long, straight, red hair and the father's hair was long and rather unkempt. He wore a short beard. I glanced at their intake history and read that the father's employment was at Sir Pizza. I thought, "The father almost surely in a near-minimum-wage job. They will have trouble with their bills. I will have to watch the charges." (This was in a time when outpatient services were seldom covered by insurance.)

The new family came in regularly for well-baby visits and immunizations. We established a friendly relationship. At the visit in March, the mother sported a deep suntan. I asked her, "How did you get such a fine suntan in the middle of winter?"

She replied, "We always spend the month of February in the family condo in Florida."

Her in-laws owned all the Sir Pizza franchises in Middle Tennessee.

I remember another family of a firstborn baby that I saw toward the end of my career. The parents were dressed very casually in faded jeans and casual shirts. The father's hair was shoulder length.

During the next several months, the baby thrived and they never missed an appointment. As usual, the family and I became friends. I knew from reviewing their chart that the father was in the music business—a common employment in the Nashville area.

We usually chatted about the latest news from the country music business. After one visit, I mentioned that Carolyn and I had recently attended a party for two of our friends on Music Row. They were celebrating their recent record that made number one on the charts.

My patient's father said, "I don't know them, but I have had six platinum records this year myself. I write for Alabama."

Don't judge a book by its cover—or a patient by his wardrobe.

Sad Times for a Pediatrician

I was in the baby business for forty years. During that time, I saw lots of babies—babies of every type and hue. I saw sick ones, well ones, big ones and small ones, happy ones and sad ones. Many sad situations stick in my memory, and victims of child abuse are to me the saddest of all.

One family stands out in my memory. I was called to the local hospital newborn nursery one evening to evaluate a baby born prematurely. My initial exam revealed a small, scrawny baby boy. He was quite underweight for his gestational age, but otherwise seemed okay. He was active and pink and had no obvious respiratory problems. It was apparent he had suffered from a lack of proper intrauterine nutrition. Even though he seemed in no immediate difficulty, I arranged a transfer to Vanderbilt neonatal service because he was likely to develop problems, such as low blood sugar, during the next several days.

I explained my actions to the baby's mother, and she seemed to take the news of the temporary loss of her baby with only minimal distress. Her live-in boyfriend seemed to be affected more severely, even though he was not the baby's father. (I thought of him as the step-boyfriend.)

A few weeks later, Vanderbilt transferred the baby back to the local hospital. I discharged the baby in a week or two, when he had attained enough weight to maintain his temperature without outside warming.

The baby kept his well-child appointments irregularly and was admitted to Vanderbilt pediatrics more than once with complaints of apnea spells. Studies revealed a bleed between the brain and skull, typical of child abuse. I reported the case to the state children's services, but somehow he remained with the mother and her live-in boyfriend, pro tem.

About eighteen months later, this mother delivered a second boy. Once again, he suffered from intrauterine malnutrition and grew poorly. At two months, I obtained x-rays of all the baby's bones and found eleven fractures in various stages of healing. Once again, I contacted children's services and this time, both boys were placed in foster care, where they thrived.

About two years later, their mother regained custody and I saw them again. After my exam, I said to the mother, "I'm really surprised you brought your boys back to see me. I thought you would never want to see me again, since I reported you twice and was responsible for moving them to foster care."

She replied, "But you are the best doctor we have ever had."

Communication/ Miscommunication

I heard an essay recently on the mechanics of communication, with the theory being that the communicator often triggers an unplanned-for response in the communicatee. The essayist is correct in his assessment that the communicator thinks about what he wants to communicate, says or writes it, and the recipient interprets what he hears or reads and flavors it with his own knowledge and prejudices of the moment. What goes out often is not what goes in. This brought to mind two examples from my practice.

Dog Bites

While rabies is common among wild animals in Middle Tennessee, it is rare in domestic animals. However, the possibility of rabies always must be considered in all animal bites. One Saturday morning, I saw a twelve-year-old boy who had been bitten by a dog that morning and had come in for a tetanus shot. The wound was trivial, but, as good medicine requires, I inquired about any rabies risk factors that might be present. "Did the dog look healthy?" I asked his father.

"Yes."

"Did the dog behave normally?"

"Yes."

"Was the attack provoked?"

"No."

Attacking unprovoked is very unusual behavior in a pet dog and raises the suspicion of possible rabies exposure. "Tell me the circumstances of the bite," I asked.

His father replied, "My son merely went into a fenced backyard to mow, and the dog ran out and bit him."

With some relief, I said, "Oh, that's a provoked attack."

He drew himself up, crossed his arms, inhaled and, in a firm voice, said, "It was not provoked! I own a lawn service and have a contract with that condominium. We had a legal right to be in the backyard!"

Upper Respiratory Infections

One day, I saw a young infant with an uncomplicated cold. After examining the baby, I sat down with the first-time mother and explained, "Your baby has a cold. You can help make her comfortable with a humidifier, some saltwater nose drops, and perhaps some Tylenol if she becomes fussy."

"Doesn't she need an antibiotic?" her mother asked.

"No. Not at this point. Antibiotics can't cure a cold, and as a matter of fact, there is no medicine that can cure this type of illness. Call me if she seems worse or you become concerned."

About an hour later, I received a frantic call from the baby's grandmother. "What's wrong with my granddaughter? My daughter told me you said she has an incurable disease! Can't you do something?"

Often what we say is not what is heard.

Pediatrics, How You Have Changed!

I was reminded while reading the paper this morning how radically pediatrics has grown and changed over my fifty years of interest in the specialty.

While I was a student and house officer, over one hundred cases of paralytic polio were admitted to Vanderbilt per year. A whole floor in the hospital was devoted to the exclusive treatment of the most severely affected patients. Iron lungs occupied most of the rooms. Without them, those patients would have died. Thanks to the vaccine, polio is a rarity—virtually wiped out in this country and much of the world. Almost every case now is caused by the vaccine, a one in several million chance. Newer vaccine regimens have even eliminated this very rare occurrence.

During my training, I saw cases of rickets, scurvy, diphtheria, pertussis, congenital syphilis, and measles to name a few. (Pertussis was just flagged by my computer's spellcheck and was not listed in my Webster's Dictionary, 2003 edition.) Almost no pediatrician trained in the last twenty years has ever seen any of these diseases, except for pertussis, which pops up very occasionally to present as a diagnostic problem for the contemporary physician. It takes an old geezer from my generation to even think of the possibility of these diseases.

And now, thanks to new vaccines, otitis media (earache) seems to be on the way to the list of diseases I label as paleopediatrics. Oh, that it will. Children with frequent episodes and persistent episodes have frustrated generation after generation of parents and pediatricians alike.

I do not fear modern pediatricians will go hungry. Childhood obesity with its accompanying long-term sequellae, attention disorders, asthma, and teenage STDs and other "modern" maladies promise to keep the pediatricians' waiting rooms full.

Medical Firsts

I was lucky to be in medical school and in training during a golden age of discovery. The beginnings or early development of virology, cardiac surgery, neonatology, the development of multiple broad-spectrum antibiotics, and the chemical basis of immunity and inheritance are some that come to mind. This was the age of rapid increases of funding for biomedical research by private foundations and by the federal government. Whether there is a connection between blossoming research and burgeoning funding is unproven, but likely.

The development and widespread use of the polio vaccine was a major accomplishment during my early medical days. Dr. John Enders developed a method of propagating the virus and Dr. Jonas Salk headed a large team of researchers who developed the first vaccine. His group developed methods of purifying the virus and then inactivating it to render it non-infectious but still a potent stimulator of antibodies in vaccine recipients. His efforts were supported by the March of Dimes, promoted by President Roosevelt, a victim of the disease.

Pressure to grow, inactivate, bottle, and distribute the new vaccine nationwide quickly came from the March of Dimes, the public, and the president. In the rush to satisfy the demand, one lot of the vaccine virus was not totally inactivated and was not detected in safety tests before release. Widespread panic resulted from the several cases of paralysis that developed as a result of the vaccine. Fortunately, most patients had developed enough immunity from earlier doses to protect them from a second or third dose containing the poorly inactivated virus.

One afternoon during my internship, I started an IV on the young grandchild of a wealthy man. He watched me start the IV and hang a bottle of fluids. He noticed the label on the bottle and asked, "Is that Cutter the same company that made the bad polio vaccine?"

"It sure is. We use Cutter fluids all over the hospital."

He pulled out a notebook and pen and wrote, "Buy Cutter."

Influenza

It seems that we may be in the beginning of a severe influenza epidemic this year. No matter what the severity of the epidemic, though, the symptoms in individual illness are often severe either way. The flu vaccine is a useful preventative, but is only effective in about two-thirds of cases. Still, it's about all we can do. The injection is virtually painless and causes few if any side effects, no matter what your friends tell you. There is little reason to avoid flu vaccine.

I spent part of my time for about thirty years as part of various teams studying vaccines. With any new vaccine, we always included a large number of control subjects, people who were given a placebo instead of the real vaccine. Sometimes the numbers and severities of side effects were more frequent in the placebo group than in the vaccine group. There is just no way to avoid that pesky placebo effect.

Years ago, in my first year of solo practice, a flu epidemic struck in December. I had been in practice less than six months, and finances were still tight. I had managed to collect enough to meet my overhead, but little was left over for me to live on.

I looked at the developing epidemic with mixed emotions. I hated to see such suffering as flu produces, but could not help but relish the thought of the increased income a flu epidemic would produce.

The epidemic became severe enough that schools over the entire county were closed early for Christmas holidays.

Shortly after Christmas, the epidemic seemed to be lessening, and schools were open once again. Within weeks, the epidemic began to worsen, and once again I faced it with mixed emotions. January seemed be hard on children but good for the bottom line.

And then came snow and ice and frigid temperatures and school closures once again. Snow recurred throughout the month, resulting in schools being closed most of January. That stopped the epidemic in its tracks. Everyone became healthy, no longer needing my services. I watched my checking account dwindle once again.

But in spite of that little setback, I survived the first year and the practice prospered for the next twenty-five years with or without influenza.

What's In a Name?

I am a Junior, and my son is a Third. That numerical designation seldom presented a problem while my son was growing up. He was a child; I am an adult. If there happened to be a reason for confusion, people called him "Little Bill." He didn't seem to mind the diminutive addition tagged on him by family members and friends. Schools were no problem. He was "Bill." I was "Bill's father."

And then came college and medical school and marriage. No name problems there. He was five-hundred-and-forty-two miles away in medical school at the University of North Carolina, and our father-son relationship was limited to telephone calls, tuition checks, and visits at holiday times.

And then came Bill's entrance into private practice. His practice of cardiology had been anchored at Baptist Hospital in Nashville, and I had patients in the newborn nursery there almost every day of the year.

And then the name thing became a problem. The Division of Medical Records wields a club over every doctor in the hospital. They examine every chart, and reject charts that have incomplete data, no matter how trivial the omission might be. Everyone had incomplete charts.

Medical Records somehow refused to acknowledge that there were two William Fleets on staff, and they seemed to put incomplete charts into either pile without thought. My charts were salted with cardiology charts, and

Bill's pile always contained charts of newborn babies. Despite repeated reminders, charts continued to be assigned randomly.

Finally, I developed a plan to solve the irritating problem. I signed my charts, "William Fleet, the Elder" and amended Bill's charts to "William Fleet, the Younger." It worked for Pliny two thousand years ago. It should work for me.

It didn't. But my problem solved itself. I retired and now I am known again as Dr. Fleet's father.

Chapter Two, Computers

Computers are alive among us. They somehow seem to have almost human traits. Most times they are quietly helpful. Sometimes they are stubbornly unyielding in their protestations at even the most innocent errors on the user's part. Sometimes they pout. They refuse to do anything—just sit unmoved by any pleas of the operator.

But I don't see how we ever lived without one.

Computers, a Love-Hate Relationship

The only thing more unreasonably stubborn than a computer is the old retired mule on our farm.

In retirement, I had to type my own correspondence, and using a typewriter proved much more difficult than I had remembered. It soon became clear that, at least for word-processing, I needed a computer.

My nephew had replaced his laptop that winter and gave me his old one as a Christmas gift (a hand-me-up.) After Christmas, it sat for a day or two, sleeping in its case waiting for the touch of a human hand. "Computers can't be too difficult. Everyone is using them all over the world, and even children operate them," I reasoned as I tentatively opened it. "This is not so hard. There's the 'On' button." I pressed it, and suddenly, the Windows logo appeared on the screen, followed by several rows of little icons. One said "My Computer" so I clicked it, assuming that "My Computer" would tell me all about MY COMPUTER. Wrong! All sorts of things appeared, none of which made any sense at all. I realized I should turn it off and buy an instruction book, but there was no "Off" button.

Finally, I called my niece for help. When she said, "Click the 'Start' icon," I realized that computers are very counterintuitive, and I was in big trouble!

Bill Gates, what have you done?

The very next day, I bought Windows or Dummies but it was far over my head. I needed Windows for Idiots. My children, grandchildren, and friends tried to help but they demonstrated maneuvers so quickly that I became totally lost after their second mouse clicks. My second trip to the computer store provided me with a new book. Its contents read, "Exercise 1: 'Start Windows'. Exercise 2: 'Left click, double click, and right click." My kind of book.

With book in hand and computer on lap, I began my cyber-education. I learned to do amazing things: to start a program; to exit a program; to minimize, restore, and maximize a window; to move a window; to left-click (both single and double); to right click; and to create a document. It was wonderful!

Soon, I became confident enough to create a spreadsheet of my income tax deductions. After three hours of intense, teeth-grinding effort, I finished a task that would have taken about a half-hour to do by hand. But I had done it on the computer! Then I set out to save it. I hit the wrong key and, in a nanosecond, the whole thing disappeared into the cyber-swamp, never to be seen or heard from again.

After about four months of using my obsolete laptop, I bought a fast, powerful desktop and slowly began to feel comfortable with the stupid, stiff-necked thing. Of course, I was on the Internet and I no longer felt guilty when "You have performed an illegal operation" appeared. RAM, ROM, megabytes, gigabytes, and megahertz rolled trippingly off my tongue (apologies to Mr. Shakespeare). A, C, and Zip drives were no longer mysteries. I knew that "defrag" had nothing to do with the Vietnam War. I knew what virus scan, firewall and spam killer do. I even become brave enough to call Technical Support a time or two.

After five years, my once-new, once-powerful, once-fast desktop had become old, weak, and slow. It had become progressively more senile day by day. It seemed that I needed a new computer. I explored buying a new Dell on the Internet. As soon as I downloaded my choices, my computer began to perform almost up to its previous standards. I renamed it "Hal."

Unfortunately, it regained its quirks in a few weeks and began to add new ones almost daily. It refused to defrag or to scandisk. It sent more and more error messages. It even began to reboot itself. Consultations with computer-competent friends convinced me that Hal was in his death throes, and I ordered the Dell. I added a one-hundred-and-sixty-nine-dollar home installation and data migration service as well.

Why can't computer techno-nerds speak English? Why "data migration"? Why not "transfer files"? Why "reboot" when everyone understands "restart"? Where did "modem" come from anyway?

I am writing this on Dell and Hal is in several pieces in the garage. Dell is brighter, faster and his graphics are sharper. He is just terrific. I delight in his presence. The joy of his addition has overcome the frustrations of adjusting to his arrival. It reminds me of bringing home a new baby.

Hal, the Final Chapter

Hal had given way to Dell, and languished alone in my workshop, awaiting his fate. I had read articles about hackers breaking into discarded computers to retrieve sensitive data even after it had been deleted. I checked with my great-nephew computer guru, John. "Oh yes," he said. "Anyone can restore files in the Recycle Bin. There's nothing to it."

"Then it would be a good idea to erase my hard drive."

He agreed.

I had saved two newspaper articles describing how to erase a hard drive. I tried both techniques. Neither worked. Another call to John produced a third method, which was unsuccessful as well. I called John a third time and asked, "What else can I do? Could I take the hard drive out and smash it with a hammer?"

He replied, "That would do it."

Screws anchored metal panels on each side of the case. It was simple to remove the panels. I opened the case and stared at a confusing collection of components. There were several circuit boards. Wires and cables were everywhere, connecting everything to everything else forming a tousled electronic maze. A transformer was attached to the back wall, and a rack holding four eight-track-tape-sized objects lay against the front wall. I saw nothing that remotely resembled a disc. Another call to John.

"It should be one of those things in the rack," he replied. Close inspection revealed that three of them opened into slots for a CD ROM, a zip disc, and a floppy disc. The fourth had to be the hard drive.

How to get it out? I unscrewed about twenty screws and removed the three unwanted components, but the hard drive refused to budge. After I removed the power pack, barking a knuckle in the process, I could see a final screw anchoring the hard drive. It was tucked under the plastic top and almost against the front panel. The front and top had to come off. How to do that? I finally noticed several almost hidden plastic clips—three on each side of the front panel. Releasing six clips simultaneously while prying off the panel required more than two hands. I solved that problem with small wooden wedges made from clothespins. Even though I had loosened both sides of the front panel, it still would not budge. Light taps and then heavier taps with a hammer were equally unsuccessful. (I had applied the following rule: don't force it, just hit it harder.) Finally, I noticed a seventh clip, which when released, allowed the front and top covers to be removed, exposing the offending little screw.

I made short work of the screw and the hard drive meekly surrendered itself into my hands. But there was no disc, just a heavy plastic and metal thing that I could not open. There was no way that I could bash it with a hammer. It was too tough.

Another call to John. I suggested, "Could I burn it?"

"Sure. Nobody could read a hard drive after that."

And so I did. I placed the hard-drive in a disposable aluminum pan and poured an entire can of charcoal lighter fluid over it.

Hal fought me at every step, even at his execution. The first match went out before it landed in the pan. The second landed on the edge of the hard drive in such a way that the burning head was exposed above the lighter fluid with the remainder beneath the surface. The paper match acted as a wick and the head burned brightly for over five minutes, refusing to light anything else. A third match landed in the lighter fluid but was doused upon landing. How can a flammable fluid put out a burning match? Hal must still have been at work. As a last resort, I played the hot flame of my propane torch over surface of the fluid. Finally, I had my fire.

For twenty minutes, I watched burning lighter fluid and an expanding circle of burning grass and listened to a crackling, popping hard drive. Even though Hal had fought me almost his entire last year, it was sad to see him go. But life must go on.

I wondered, "What wine goes best with barbecued hard drive?"

Not Simple Enough for an Adult to Use

Last winter I borrowed a four-DVD set about great characters of the Old Testament from one of our associate pastors. I thought the DVDs might be fodder for a series of Sunday School lessons. We rotate teachers from our class, and I teach four weeks a year. My new computer can play DVDs, but I had not yet attached speakers. That would be a simple task— or so I had thought.

However, I have yet to find anything about computers to be simple.

My new computer has three triple outlets, variously labeled with something related to sound. I plugged the speakers into one of the outlets and proceeded to play a DVD. No sound issued. Even more unsettling, a window appeared that said, "You have the wrong area code for this DVD." Why "area code"? I wasn't making a long distance call. At least I did not think I was. Not only did I not know how to change the area code, but I had no idea which area code I should use. It seemed that the DVD set must return to the church.

The Christmas season is a thief of time. (I think I should apologize to Mr. Shakespeare here.) Helping to prepare three gallons of seafood gumbo for two family get-togethers, trimming the Christmas tree, helping decorate the house, and manning our daughter's table at the Martin Senior Center's first bazaar consumed a lot of time in addition to my usual busy-work retirement duties. As a result, the DVD set lay fallow beside my computer. It could be returned after Christmas.

Most years, I bought Carolyn something and that was all of my Christmas shopping; she did the rest. This year was different. Carolyn's pain problems limit her walking and standing, so I did a significant part of our Christmas shopping.

One of my tasks was to buy a DVD player for a grandchild. While standing in line to pay, I suddenly realized that for sixty dollars, I could have my own DVD player. Forget the computer. I could use the TV! I came home with two DVD players. I unpacked mine and hooked it into our TV—a simple task.

I never learn. Nothing electronic is ever simple. I got no sound. I got no picture. I got nothing. I was stymied. I would have to read the unintelligible owner's manual—a sentence of thirty minutes of confusing, poorly written English interspersed with Spanish, French, and Japanese (or is it Chinese?). I thought, "My grandchildren from Georgia will be here in four days. They can hook it up." And so, I just let the player and its owner's manual lay dormant, awaiting the touch of an expert hand. The day they arrived, I asked seventeen-year-old Jacob to fix my DVD player, and in five minutes it was happily playing DVDs.

The Georgia grandchildren left for home on Christmas Eve. As they were packing, Carolyn asked fifteen-year-old Leigh if she could make her new cellphone ring louder, something we had failed to accomplish. Within two minutes, not only had Leigh increased the ring volume, but also had demonstrated all the choices for ring sounds and had programmed the one Carolyn liked best.

Carolyn asked, "How did you know how to do that?"

Jacob replied, "Grandmother, we were born knowing how."

It's Just a Little Computer Chip

Last fall we almost wrecked our car and Lynne's back porch.

Our son and his wife recently moved into their new home, Lynne's dream house. Everything is just so, and the whole house follows Federal architecture to the letter (except that it does have running water and electricity.)

Carolyn and I delivered some stepstools and tomatoes that Sunday afternoon, and when we tried to leave, the car refused to start. We tried jumper cables without success and were left with only one alternative: a tow truck. A call to AAA produced a tow truck in about an hour.

The truck was the type that carried the disabled car on its cargo-bed rather than towing it behind. The operator lowered the bed to make a ramp and our car slowly crawled upward, pulled by a cable winch. All went well until it was almost in place for transport, when CRACK! The towing ring under the front bumper broke free. Our car backed down the ramp, slowly at first—and then faster and faster down the ramp and faster and faster still, down a slope, directly toward the new patio and porch.

Our wiry tow truck operator dashed for the car, flung open the door, and oblivious to the risk of being run over, dove in and braked to a stop only feet from the house. He reattached the cable, and reloaded the car without further incident.

Early Monday morning, our garage called. I described our problem. They went to work, starting with the most likely defect, the starter motor. After an hour or so, they called with their verdict: the problem was only a defective little computer chip in my ignition key. But while working on the starter, they noticed a water pump leak, an omen of sudden failure in the near future. I okayed its replacement and asked them to change the oil and rotate the tires since our car was already in the shop. About 4 pm, they called. We needed twenty dollars for a water pump pulley; we okayed that as well. Since they couldn't get the pulley Monday, they would need to keep the car another day.

Okay.

On Tuesday, they called. While rotating the tires, they found that we needed to have the brakes replaced. Since this is a safety item, there was nothing else to do but okay that as well. New wiper blades rounded out the repairs.

Upon picking up our car, I found that the faulty little computer chip ended up costing $694.70.

Some little computer chip! And it hadn't even been fixed!

An Analog Person in a Digital Age

As is my custom, I sat down at my computer just after breakfast. I checked my email and printed one message. The printer worked fine. Later, I tried to print my weekly column for my hard copy files, and my printer refused to print. Nor would it copy. I didn't try to scan anything. It always takes about a half-hour of false moves for me to do that.

I looked at the tiny copier screen and it said, "Remove and check cartridge." I did that, though I could see nothing to check. I replaced the cartridge, washed the ink off my fingers, and restarted the printer; same message. New cartridge, same message. A sharp blow to the printer top, same message. My last hope was the dreaded technical support.

I contacted the manufacturer and, for nineteen dollars, received this message, "Clean the printer head with a swab and hot water. If this fails to correct your problem you will need a new printer head."

I thought, "Nothing as simple as hot water would cure anything digital," and I was right.

Off to the computer store I went.. I walked into the store and accosted the youngest salesclerk I could find. I assumed the younger the advisor, the more about electronics he knew. He confirmed my suspicion that it would take about a hundred dollars to replace the head. We toured the printer aisle. There was row after row of printers that printed, copied, scanned, and faxed, all cheaper than repairing my old one. I picked one on sale.

Fifty-three years ago, I assembled a Hi-Fi system from piles of wire, resistors, capacitors, vacuum tubes, and transformers. It worked on first try—well, second try. I had forgotten to connect the cable between the amplifier and the speaker at first. But it played records faultlessly for years without hiccup. It still worked when I sold it in a yard sale. I figured I should be able to install the printer. After all, I only had to connect two wires and the job would be done.

And so I began. I finished unpacking and searched out installation instructions. They were printed in English, French, Spanish, and Portuguese. Connecting the two cords properly went without a hitch. Then began my trouble. I noticed a message in Portuguese scrolling across the half-Band-Aid-sized screen. I thought, "It shouldn't be problem to switch it to English," but I was wrong. I pressed an arrow button again and again, and only Portuguese appeared. I thought, "Maybe I bought a Portuguese machine and will have to enroll in Portuguese lessons." Not to be deterred, back to the owner's manual I went. After a few false starts, I found a way to select English. I felt a warm glow. I had overcome another digital challenge.

Now I had to install ink cartridges. I stuck them in the holes provided, and they promptly fell out. There was no instruction on how to install the inky things. Only after multiple attempts was I able to install them properly.

Finally, I could print.

We are in the digital age. No more analog that lasts and lasts and performs without complaint. It seems that digital is only semi-permanent—more disposable than fixable. We operate on the idea of, "Don't fix it. Buy another." And then disposing of the old ones can be a problem. But we can't live without them no matter how frustrating they can be. We are trapped in the digital age.

I'm too old to be digital. It may be less a blessing and more a curse. We super senior citizens need super-simple electronics.

Electronics, Reluctantly

I have expounded upon my travails in installing a new printer for my computer. I am proud to say I have now adapted to it. When I obey its English commands, it performs. I do wish it were not quite so bossy. Compared to my previous printers, it is faster and more convenient if I am suitably submissive.

Computers, I've figured out. TVs, not so much. We have two dens, one upstairs where Carolyn has her nest and one downstairs where I hang out. We have a TV in each. Carolyn watches hers upstairs; I watch mine downstairs. Seldom do we watch the same program unless it happens to be an important athletic event. Both sets are analog.

We began to notice that Carolyn's TV picture is not as sharp as it once was, and that for a few minutes after startup, the color had a faded yellowish tint. We surmised that the old TV was in its death throes and we began to think about a new TV. Of course, it would be digital and we could pay the cable company their surcharge for a high definition modem. (I think modem is the correct term for the little box with the yellow and blue lights.)

I dug out my Consumer's Reports article on TVs and turned immediately to the ratings. All that technical stuff is boring and tends to go over my head. We picked the brand and model number that seemed best for us, and began to shop. To no surprise, our choice models were no longer available. We were left flying blind once again in the land of the all-powerful digital electronics.

Finally we chose one and brought it home. Our grandson installed it as best he could, but we needed a new modem from the cable company. A competent, friendly installation specialist arrived on time at our house and proceeded to connect our new TV to the cable so that we could see things in high definition.

The picture was grand. I could count the blades of grass on the football field. But the sound was terrible no matter how we adjusted it. I had read that the sound in the modern sets was suspect, and our new TV certainly verified that observation.

❦

So, it was back to the mall. We came home with two new sets. (I couldn't resist the call of HD.)

The cable guy comes next week. I can hardly wait.

Maybe I'll buy a new cellphone. I can learn to do Facebook and tweet and texting and take pictures and no telling what else.

I feel so twenty-first century.

Another Crisis in Cyberland

It was an ordinary day, my usual time to check my email and visit my usual computer stops. But it didn't remain ordinary for very long. I attempted to read my email. I couldn't connect on first try or second try. I knew just what to do. I called my Internet provider for my usual remedy—a quick fix of my modem via the telephone. This time, it failed to fix my problem. I talked with their first line of defense in cyberland, and it soon became obvious my problem was beyond his capabilities. It seemed to be in my computer, not in the cable. He handed me off to a second technical support person with whom I met with the same lack of success.

On to India. Those guys can do anything except vocal communication. Southern Indian and Southern American do not mesh. Finally, we resorted to a private chatroom, and communications improved immeasurably. My guy, Astoush, and I chatted a short while and he quickly diagnosed my problem. I had forgotten that Microsoft's free maintenance program expired after about two years and so my computer had not had its innards scrubbed at least that long. Astoush proceeded to clean out hundreds of useless temporary files and other trash gumming up my computer—for a charge of over three hundred dollars. But that fee includes two years of routine maintenance plus any technical support necessary during that time.

With my computer humming along faster than I had remembered I tried to write a column. No luck. Microsoft Word refused to behave. It wouldn't do anything I asked.

And then I remembered. That program was a leased service, and my lease had run out. I renewed my lease and tried to install it. No luck. Right in the middle of installation it stopped and demanded I remove the old program. I fumbled and fumed for almost an hour until I managed to comply. But now the new program had disappeared in mid-instillation and I had no idea how to resurrect it. I tried several remedies without success. Finally I resorted to restoring the computer to an earlier date—a seemingly foolproof remedy. But not in my hands.

My computer hung up part way to restoring and refused to budge. I was stymied. I did what I should have done earlier. I called Astoush. He was very patient and understanding as he explained how I had completely fouled up the installation. I was one step away from completely crashing my computer. It took over four hours to diagnose the problem and fix it.

At the end of our encounter Astoush said, "Don't ever try to fix anything again for two years."

Cyber Monday

Whew! Never again! I have had my fill of Cyber Monday. I managed to avoid Gray Thursday and Black Friday and whatever they called Saturday or Sunday. Cyber Monday slipped up on me.

My younger daughter called on her cellphone this morning asking me to buy tickets on line for a play at the Tennessee Performing Arts Center.

"Dad, I'm on my way to work and I am trying to buy tickets from TPAC. I have been on hold for forever. Would you buy the tickets for me online? I have a meeting in a few minutes."

"Sure."

"I'll walk you through it. First, access their website."

"I have it."

"Click 'Tickets.'"

"Done. I get a message saying I am in the waiting room and in line to buy tickets."

"Good. I need two tickets to Catch Me If You Can."

"Okay."

I began to receive messages every forty-eight seconds saying I was in line to access TPAC. I received repeats of the original message in the same irritating, syrupy voice on the telephone saying, "Your message is very important to us." I don't see much improvement in robotic messages asking me to wait. Both are irritating robotic stop signs to progress.

By then, my daughter had signed off as she entered a meeting at work. I continued to wait, staring at the screen reassuring me that TPAC computers were busy and I was in line to make my purchase. Finally, after about twenty minutes, the screen changed to ticket sales.

I began to establish an account. It seemed to take about two minutes to progress to each new information box. TPAC must have either too few computers or old, out-of-date computers, because every step seemed to take forever to accomplish. It was click on a box, wait as long as a typical wait at the light on Old Hickory Boulevard/Franklin Road intersection, then click on the next box, wait another traffic light, and do it again and again.

Toward the end of the sluggish data acquisition, there appeared a box labeled "Donation $8.40." I had used up all my patience by then, so I let it go through. It was worth the money to be able to finish.

I clicked "Submit" and, of course, nothing happened. After waiting through two lights, I assumed I was done and clicked out of the TPAC website. If I hadn't finished, I had at least quit. I hope my grandson and his wife wouldn't be too disappointed if they didn't get tickets.

Addendum: I later printed an automated email from TPAC saying my order would be mailed the next day. I'm so proud. I did it. But never again on a Cyber Monday.

Chapter 3, Seasons

I had a friend who moved to Southern California some years ago. When he returned to Nashville, I asked him how he liked it. He said he didn't care for it. The weather was unchangeably fine—warm breezes, cloudless skies, infrequent rain. He missed the seasons.

I think I would miss seasons as well. With seasons, I have something to complain about the year round.

Weather

Where were you the last time we had storms? Did you watch the fronts go through? Did you tire of weather-related time-filling by all three networks? I could not unglue my eyes from the TV screen or loosen my hand on the TV remote. I just sat there dumbly, watching storm cells move in their stately manner across the screen and through my neighborhood.

Were you just a little bit disappointed, or were you merely relieved that the tornado gods smiled once again and steered them away from Brentwood? I have never been in a tornado, and hope never to be in one. I have seen the results of a few. I much prefer the vicarious experience of seeing them on TV.

My parents grew up in Oklahoma, part of tornado alley. My paternal grandparents had a storm cellar just off their kitchen door, just beyond the cistern. It was mostly beneath ground level, made of concrete with a concrete floor. The walls were lined with shelves for home-canned food storage. The concrete floor was the ideal place to cool watermelons since the temperature remained unchanging in the 50s. I loved to play in the cool cellar during the summertime.

I saw no tornadoes there, but did once experience a dust storm. I remember the high-boiling, dirty cloud reaching across the horizon, slowly moving toward us. The sun dimmed to deep twilight and the air cooled noticeably as the cloud engulfed us in a gritty world of dust. It frightened this five-year-old boy out of his wits.

I spent two days as a relief worker in East Nashville after the tornado in 1998. Every person I met on my rounds delivering food and water was most appreciative of my efforts. Rubberneckers elicited a different reaction among the victims. I was talking with one lady after my food delivery one day, when a police cruiser crept by.

She stepped onto the street, stopping the cruiser. She asked, "Are you on duty?"

He replied, "No, just looking."

She stood straight-backed, head erect, crossed her arms, stared at him, and spat out, "Then just get the hell out of here!"

A tornado leveled about two-thirds of my hometown in Mississippi some years ago, years after I had established my home in Brentwood. I visited my parents about a week after the damage was done. Mercifully, nobody was injured.

There are two things about the tornado I remember. All five of the churches in the town were destroyed but not one of the three liquor stores was touched. I don't know if there is a moral in that or not.

There was lot after lot where the houses were totally destroyed, and only a toilet bolted to the foundation slab remained. I decided that if I am ever in a tornado, I would go to the bathroom and sit on the toilet.

From what I have seen, tornados are powerful, destructive things. Let us hope we continue to watch them on TV and not in person.

Our First Snow

Midway through my breakfast today, I glanced out of the window and there, falling out of the sky, was snow. Flakes were very small and few in number, but nevertheless it was snow. It wasn't sleet or rain. It was snow. I admit it was light enough that it would take a week or more to accumulate enough to cover the ground. But still, it was snow.

I once became excited to see snow. Even this puny performance would engender hopes of school closures and sledding in my childhood and youth. But after living in Pennsylvania, Washington, D.C., and Sweden, snow now fails to stir my enthusiasm.

I grew up in the Deep South where temperatures in the low 40s were unusual. Water pipes were laid on the surface under houses, and the rare temperatures below freezing resulted in frozen pipes. Any snow was signal for school closures and celebrations among the children. I remember snow accumulations of an inch or more only twice before I left for college. Neither snowfall accumulated enough for sledding, but then, nobody had a sled nor were there hills to slide down.

We saw enough snow in Sweden to last me a lifetime. There was snow on the ground from December through April. By winter's end, streets were defined by head-high piles of snow thrown up by daily snowplowing. Children skated on rinks created by flooding flat places on lawns. Cars navigated on snow-covered streets and highways almost as fast as on dry pavement.

I remember seeing an elderly lady walking along a snow-clad Swedish sidewalk pushing a chair on long sled runners. I told Carolyn, "What a great idea. She has a great way to avoid a fall and a broken hip." When she reached the top of a hill she gave her chair a shove, hopped on the sled runners, and zoomed down the hill.

After over fifty years living in Nashville, I find that snow has regained a bit of its mystique. I like to see the ground covered with a pristine layer of fresh snow, but I am glad it seldom comes and interferes with my life. I don't miss it, but wouldn't it be great if we had a white Christmas?

Winter Doldrums

It's January and cold. I sit at the breakfast table slurping down my oatmeal and raisins. The temperature has been below freezing for a week; my electricity and gas bills will be out of sight this month. Snow is on its way.

The ground is frozen; the bird bath is frozen; birds are fluffed up in the cold; our pansies are sickly, all limp and pale; my truck probably won't start; and all I have to look forward to is February—and you know February. It's the August of winter—better experienced somewhere else than Middle Tennessee. Maybe I will spend a few weeks with one of my grandsons in Scottsdale, Arizona. It was sixty-one degrees there yesterday. But then, I would have to play golf every day.

And I have to go to the grocery. I really do. We're out of milk and bread. Can't survive the rigors of winter without milk and bread. I will drag myself to the store, crowded though it will be. I hope I can find a cart. If I were a burglar, today would be an ideal day to practice my trade. The entire police force is probably shopping as well.

Mid-afternoon.

I survived the grocery store. Lunch of soup and cheese and apple is over. And the mail arrived. Hidden in the paper spam was my first seed catalog of the year. It is filled with beautiful pictures of flowers and vegetables screaming, "Plant me! Plant me!" Perhaps the catalog is the light at the end of the tunnel, or the first robin of spring, or maybe the sign that soon there will be dirt under my fingernails.

If seed catalogs come, can spring be far behind? (Apologies to Percy Shelley.)

Winter Doldrums II

Winter now is upon us, and we expect the temperature to fasten its grip on us in Middle Tennessee for many weeks, mixing icy cold with slightly warmer days. Snow is not a regular feature here, but when it comes, it comes as a major nuisance.

Another facet of winter is the waning light. Days become shorter with great regularity until almost Christmastime, when they begin to lengthen a bit each day. During our year's stay in Stockholm, Sweden it was the darkness that affected us more than the cold and snow—though we had plenty of both.

Darkness there became evident in late autumn and was profound in December. The sun shone brightly only a total of eight hours for the entire month of December. The remainder of the month was either cloudy or snowing. Our two-year-old forgot what sunshine was and complained about the light hurting his eyes on the single sunny day of the month.

By Christmas, we experienced only four hours of daylight a day. Daylight was of twilight intensity, not strong enough to eliminate the need for artificial lights indoors and out.

We in the United States have a wide variation of winter weather, from the warmth of Florida to the cold of North Dakota. I will close this chapter with the story of a North Dakotan farmer told to me by a colleague. I trust it is true. He insisted it was, and since he has died, who's to challenge it?

Sam spent each January on one of the resort islands of the Caribbean basking in the sunshine on the beach. (He must have had an independent fortune to afford such luxury as a pediatrician.)

One evening, he noticed a new face in the hotel dining room. They nodded to each other and went their own ways. The next morning at breakfast, the stranger approached Sam and began a conversation: "Pardon me, sir but I noticed you here yesterday and wonder if I could ask you a question."

"Sure. What is it?"

"I'm a rancher from North Dakota and, as you know, I arrived here yesterday. My brother and I own a large cattle ranch. We are suffering the worst winter in memory. I am fed up with getting up before dawn, fighting sub-zero temperatures and high winds, hauling hay, breaking ice on water troughs, and rescuing downed cattle. It became so bad I had to take a break. I called a travel agent and told her to put me on the first flight out of there going south and to keep scheduling flights south until I landed in someplace warm.

My question is, 'Where am I?'"

Weather, Reprise

Written four months ago, just after the floods. Somehow I didn't have the heart to send it for publication until now.

I'm sitting at my computer on Sunday morning, hearing an occasional thunderclap and listening to rain pour down. I'm fearful every minute that a power surge will come and totally fry my new computer. It's so new that I am just now becoming somewhat comfortable with its new program. I think it is a relative of Hal.

Uh-oh. The lights flickered, but my computer is okay. Maybe Hal Junior can weather the storm. And what a storm! Yesterday, I saw squall line after squall line progressing across the TV screen and through our yard, dumping over six inches of rain on the neighborhood. Today, the rain continues with over two inches only this morning—and rain persists. The TV is out. The Internet is out. Email is out. We are stuck in. Nowhere to go anyhow. Nothing to do when we get there—and we are out of bread.

Rain pours down, our creek is flooding, roads and yards are underwater, and some of our best friends were evacuated this morning when the swollen Little Harpeth River threatened their houses. Even the church is closed. No services today. Only the second time in the forty-six years I have been attending there that it's closed on Sunday. But so far, Hal keeps chugging along, and I do, too.

What's behind all this severe weather, anyway? Can't be global warming. We had one of the most severe winters on record. But weather is one thing; climate is another. And we can't seem to do a thing about either one.

I dread to see my garden. My poor tomato plants took a beating in the recent cold snap and had just begun to thrive—and now this. I'm glad I had no seeds in the ground. If I had, there would be beans and peas and squash and okra coming up everywhere.

Pity the poor farmer. With drought, cold, and now flood rains, he must be in early stages of depression. (Advice to non-farmers: Do not mention to your farmer friends the Bible quote, "God makes rain fall on the just and the unjust." Their sense of humor is a bit thin just now.)

Distinct seasons are one thing, but this year so far is something extraordinary. But I do like to have seasons.

Springtime

The equinox has passed. The stores are full of flowers and candy and bunnies. Spring is almost here.

Winter is over. Maybe. Pray it is. I have had enough of cold and snow and icy roads. I want to hang up my wooly coat and return the snow shovel to the barn where it belongs. I am ready for spring, for warm days, for breezy days.

It's time for short sleeves and short pants, maybe even to sweat a little. It's time for spring.

Forsythias are clothed in yellow, pear trees in pink. Daffodils nod, all shades of yellow; crocus and pansies cover beds with color. Tulip bulbs begin to bloom. Dogwoods promise blooms tomorrow. Roses and burning bushes and blackberries grow baby leaves.

Yes, spring is here. Or maybe not. Too often, cold snaps bring us back to reality. The calendar says it's spring; the weather today says it's spring; but even though we hate to admit it, we may have other winters to endure. There are dogwood winter, blackberry winter, and others. Cold refuses to give up just yet.

But today there were showers in the morning, cloudless skies, and warmth this afternoon. No matter that we may have other winters to endure; more frost to bear. I'm celebrating spring today. I put on a polo shirt. I bought tomato plants and potting soil.

I ate a Baskin Robbins ice cream cone.

I pulled out my mower.

It wouldn't start.

I tried my tiller.
It wouldn't start.
Where did I store that kite?

Summertime

We are having summer doldrums with a vengeance this year. It seems to have been uncomfortably hot for months, or maybe years. I have trouble remembering when it wasn't almost unbearable. But then, my memory isn't so great anymore.

But I do remember summers in my childhood. The Mississippi delta country is hot and humid from May to October. The land is flat, interspersed with sluggish bayous and a few boggy swamps. It is ideal for crops and snakes and deer and bugs. Mosquitoes are an every-summer plague. Nobody ventures out into the hot humid night in summertime. The air is alive with large, fat mosquitoes that fly in mass attacks on any hapless human who dares to go outside after sundown.

My great uncle swore he saw a small child carried off by four average-sized mosquitoes one summer evening. (Of course, Uncle Robert was prone to exaggerate a bit. There may have been more than four.)

People had two choices in summertime: to stay indoors and swelter or to go outside and become mosquito bait and swelter. Open screen-covered doors and windows provided ineffective cooling and imperfect protection against marauding mosquitoes, but that was about all the cooling we had.

Every August ,we enjoyed relief from heat, humidity, and insect life. We visited our ancestral home in Oklahoma. I loved my grandparents and cousins, and especially loved the weather.

Days were hot—often in the 90s with strong, steady winds every day. The humidity was low, and though the sun was hot, the wind and the low humidity made daytime living tolerable and a welcomed relief from Mississippi.

Oklahoma nights were almost unbelievable. Temperatures cooled, winds moderated into a gentle breeze, and not a single mosquito could be found. We children played hide and seek, caught fireflies, and spent lots of time lying on a quilt watching shooting stars and identifying constellations in the inky black night sky.

Oklahoma time spawned memories still vivid to this day: playing with cousins, eating things Grandma cooked for me just because I liked them, going on errands with Grandpa, sitting on a wooden box in the back of his two-seater car, riding Grandpa's horse, and eating strawberries out of the garden.

But the best part of every visit was lying on a quilt, feeling a cool breeze caress my skin, and looking up at the stars.

"Lawnmower" is a Four-Letter Word

I installed a first-class croquet court, in my backyard, some ten years ago. I bought an expensive reel-type mower to cut the Tifton Bermuda grass to the required quarter-inch height. The mower was a load to operate, but did a good job. Over the years, it cut less and less well until it became obvious its blade needed to be sharpened and adjusted. I called Sears.

"We will have to send it to Chattanooga for that."

"How long will it take to get it back?"

"Maybe a month. Maybe more."

I had a problem. The court needs to be cut at least twice a week. Now I would be without a mower for at least a month, maybe more. What to do? My best buddy, Bob, had the answer. He had an old twenty-inch walk-behind mower he no longer used. In fact, it hadn't been started in three years. He assured me, "It always starts on the third pull." I accepted his gift gratefully. Though it couldn't cut low enough for proper play, it could control the grass.

Once I had it home, I began the mower's rehabilitation. I dumped the old gas, changed the oil, and replaced the spark plug and the deteriorated air filter. A friendly pat upon its carburetor completed my renovation.

Then came the moment of truth—would it start? It did! On the third pull! Just as Bob said! Who would have believed it? I cut my court. It looked good, but the grass was too long for play. No matter. The pressure was off. I could maintain it in a holding mode until my reel mower came back.

The court needed to be mowed five days later. I hauled out Bob's mower. Three pulls on the starter rope produced nothing. Four, five, six, seven, eight pulls were no better. I bent over the mower, panting and sweating with curses coursing through my mind.

After I regained my breath and my composure, I tried again. Same result. The saner part of my brain took over. I took the mower to our local lawnmower shop.

"We can work on your mower in about a week. We will call you when it's done." That was not good news.

Time passed, grass grew, anxiety grew; there was nothing I could do.

Finally, came a call. "Your mower is ready." I dashed down to the lawnmower shop and retrieved my rusty old hand-me-down. Once home, it refused to start.

Another trip to the lawnmower shop. One pull by the mechanic produced a satisfying vroom, vroom, vroom.

I took the mower home. It refused to start. Pull after pull produced only a depressing putt, putt—not a single vroom.

I needed that mower. Back to the lawnmower shop.

"I can't get it started."

"Weren't you here yesterday?"

"That's right."

"Let's see what we can find."

He pulled the starter cord and, guess what—vroom, vroom, vroom.

Home again. Unloading once again. Pulling produced putts. No vrooms, not a single one. The mower had won! There was no way I was going to take it back to the lawnmower shop. It would be just too embarrassing to report to the mechanic that my mower hated me. I was not going to take it to counseling, either.

I solved my mower's attitude problem. I slipped it into a nearby yard sale. So much for you, buddy.

What to do now? buy a new mower, of course. I went to WalMart. Where else could I find a cheaper mower than at WalMart? I bought one, not the bottom of the line, but next to it. I debated buying such a cheap mower, but it wouldn't be doing heavy-duty work. The Brigs and Stratton motor convinced me that at least it should start.

It didn't—not a single vroom.

So, another long trek to WalMart to return the wretched thing.

"Is there any gas in the mower?" the clerk in customer service cooed.

"Well, yes, there is."

"We can't accept mowers with gas in them. It's against the fire code. You'll have to empty it before I can accept it for return. Take it directly out the nearest door. The fire marshal would close us down if he found you in the store with gas in your tank."

What to do? I lived a good twenty-five minutes from the store. Taking it home, emptying the tank, and returning it to WalMart would take most of the afternoon. Aha! I'll dump it here. I rolled the mower out and proceeded around the store, trying to be invisible. I finally found a storm drain behind the huge building at the back edge of the parking lot. The drain accepted my pint of gas without complaint or explosion. So much for you, Mr. Fire Marshal!

I tiptoed out of the parking lot and back into the store. Finally, I had my refund.

What to do now? Forget WalMart. I bought one at the lawnmower shop and hoped they didn't recognize me. I paid more, but I got a better mower.

Now I have a shiny new mower that is guaranteed to start within three pulls, and it has yet to let me down—but it is very early in the season.

A Special Halloween

About twenty years ago, Matthew, a patient, and I went trick-or-treating. We joined the several young spooks knocking on doors. But we were a bit different from the preschool and elementary school-age spooks up and down the neighborhood. I was about sixty, and Matthew was about twenty.

Matthew was a special patient of mine and a special person as well. Matthew had a rare in-born malady that resulted in very poor lung function, a weak heart, and significant developmental delay. Children with his syndrome usually die before age thirteen. Mostly because of his parent's exceptional care, Matthew was alive at twenty. He and his parents had dropped by our house for a short visit before going out for Matthew's share of candy.

I suggested I take Matthew around our neighborhood for some of the spoils of the evening. As we set out on our rounds, I instructed Matthew, "When someone answers the door say, 'Trick or treat,' and hold out your bag. Then say, 'Thank you."

At the first house, I rang the doorbell, and when the door opened, Matthew remained mute. After a minute or two, he held out his bag and the owner rewarded him with candy. No thank-you was evident.

As we left I reminded Matthew, "Remember. Say, 'Trick or treat' and hold out your bag and say, 'Thank you.'" At the next house, he forgot his lines again, but held out his bag. At every house, the same thing. No words. A bag produced. Candy. No thank-you.

Toward the end of our block, Matthew became bolder, entered a few houses uninvited, and shook hands with everyone there. (Matthew was very big on handshakes.)

We finished our rounds with a bag full of candy and not a single "trick or treat" or "thank you" uttered.

The next day at church services, Matthew and his parents walked past us as we sat in our accustomed pew. Matthew leaned over toward me and said softly, "Trick or treat."

Working on Christmas

I never minded working on Christmas. It was such a change from the days leading up to the big day. The few weeks before Christmas were always hectic. Our waiting room and appointment book were overflowing. Pleas and even a few demands for the "pink medicine" echoed throughout the office. Everyone wanted his or her child well for Christmas.

Christmas Day was different. There was an eerie quiet in suburbs and city. Nobody was about. Stores were closed. Traffic lights blinked at empty streets. I had the whole city to myself.

Even on Christmas there was work to do. I returned a few calls. That there were only a few calls was a welcomed change. There were a few patients left in hospitals, and there were a few children who needed to be seen that day even though it was Christmas. I much preferred to see those few children in my office rather than send them to a hospital emergency department where they would be exposed to a waiting room filled with patients, some of whom would be contagious and some of whom might be belligerent.

I usually made hospital rounds first. There were only a few children in the hospital and often a few in newborn nurseries. I always made an effort to discharge every one possible on this special day.

Usually there were a few patients waiting for me in the parking lot when I arrived at the office. I opened up, pulled charts, and began to see patients. Usually, I got to hold and admire Christmas dolls and trucks, and later in my career, electronics.

Christmas was usually a short workday. There were few patients in hospitals, and few patients were sick enough—or their parents were concerned enough—to require an office visit. Except for the telephone, my workday usually was done by noon.

Christmas was a rewarding day, a slow day, a day to feel necessary, and a day to feel genuinely appreciated. It was a day to make me glad to be a pediatrician.

Christmas, Full Circle

Our son and his family were in North Carolina four Christmases ago. Our two daughters were having Christmas with their in-laws, as well. We had our Christmas with a tree, three children, their three spouses, and eight grandchildren on the twentieth. As usual, there was a flurry of unwrapping, unboxing, and shouts of thanks. Most gifts seemed to be appreciated.

Christmases have changed over our forty-eight years of marriage. We celebrated our first Christmas alone together with a tiny tree and token gifts. (I was in medical school. We lived on Carolyn's meager salary, help from my family, and a little money from my part-time job.)

By our third Christmas, we had a baby beginning to crawl. A tiny tree on a table seemed to be the thing to do again. And it was all we could afford. Token gifts again were the thing; a twenty-dollar bracelet and a landscape print stretched our budget. Then two more babies came; income improved, our tree became bigger, our gifts more expensive.

For years we celebrated the day the way almost everyone does. Carolyn and I gave each other expensive clothes and jewelry. We had a big tree. There were lots of presents for the children, lots of food, and visits by the grandparents.

And then we became grandparents ourselves. We visited grandchildren on Christmas Day, and they visited us Christmas night.

Since the big gift opening time was in the morning and the grandchildren came for supper, we decided to buy a tabletop artificial tree. The children and grandchildren set up a howl. "We always have a big tree, a real tree. I don't like that little fake tree." We persisted. They adjusted.

Christmas was different four years ago. All our children and grandchildren were at their other families' homes. Carolyn and I had decided to limit the amount of our gifts to each other and give the extra money to charities.

On Christmas morning we were alone, with our little tree and with our token gifts, the way our early Christmases were.

We liked it that way.

The Twelfth Day of Christmas

The children are gone. The grandchildren are gone, along with their three dogs. No more nieces or nephews or great-nieces or great-nephews at our dinner table for several days. Christmas celebrations are definitely over.

Christmas is always busy. There were thirty-six at our niece's and nephew's house on Christmas Eve, fifteen on Christmas night at our house, and we fed seventeen for supper on the twenty-sixth.

Carolyn is the dessert chef for our extended family. For our extended Christmas, she made four chocolate chess pies, two fudge pies, one pecan pie, one jam cake, one double chocolate cake, and three éclair cakes. She also stirred up a few dozen home-baked cookies for the younger ones. One of the children looked over the desert table and asked, "Is that all?" It was enough.

I ate leftover desserts for almost two weeks after Christmas Day. At lunch on Sunday (January sixth, the twelfth day of Christmas), I finished the last dessert, a slice of double chocolate cake. Christmas was finally and officially over, escorted out in a high-calorie double chocolate finale.

On Christmas night, our extended family gathers at our house. We serve seafood gumbo and French bread and leftover deserts. We once had a sit-down dinner with rib roast, scalloped oysters, ham, and an assortment of vegetables. Gumbo was better—less last minute work. This year, our children and grandchildren exchanged presents and ate gumbo on the twenty-sixth.

Carolyn and I start gumbo several days before Christmas. A beef stock signals the beginning of our preparation. Over the ensuing days, we add a variety of ingredients to the pot. I dice onions and celery and other vegetables, and the day we serve gumbo, I peel the shrimp— ten pounds this year. It takes a lot of shrimp for over six gallons of gumbo, but it is worth every little decapod crustacean for the taste they impart.

And so, Christmas is over for another year. Our children are back at work, grandchildren are in school, and the house is beginning to resemble its pre-holiday appearance.

And it's time to regain my own post-holiday appearance. I need to lose a few pounds.

An Unexpected Christmas Present

Finding an appropriate Christmas present for Carolyn is always difficult for me. It has become even more difficult since we have agreed not to spend a lot for the presents. This year seemed to be different.

Over the past four months, we had received unsolicited calls from three roofing companies with the same story: "We are in the neighborhood roofing a house and noticed your roof has hail and wind damage. Since we are already in the neighborhood, we can give you a special price."

I am extremely leery of such unsolicited offers after hearing and reading about home repair scams foisted on unsuspecting homeowners. They seem to be targeted to older residents (and we certainly fit that category.) I refused each offer.

After the third call, we became a bit uneasy about the condition of our roof. Could it be that we really do need a new roof? Maybe. With that disturbing thought in mind, I called our insurance agent. I thought that though our roof is about fifteen years old it is a "twenty-five-year roof" and if we do need a new roof, insurance might help a bit.

An adjuster came out promptly. He and his assistant tromped around our roof, then came down and announced, "You do have significant hail and wind damage. You need a new roof." He also suggested a roofing company that was competent and did work for a fair price.

A representative of the roofing company came our promptly, thumped across our roof, and pronounced, "You need a new roof. I will send you an estimate next week."

Next week brought unhappy news. The estimate was over seventeen thousand dollars. I gulped twice and wondered how I could tie a red ribbon on our chimney Christmas Eve night. We sent the roofer's estimate and the adjuster's report to our insurer and waited nervously to see how much, if any, they would pay.

Within a week, a check for fourteen thousand dollars arrived.

I thought, "I guess I'll have to find Carolyn a Christmas present after all."

Christmas Gift

It's Christmastime, a time of shopping, of wrapping, of Christmas cards, of giving gifts, of receiving gifts, of Santa Claus, of parties, of fellowship, of good times, and of sometimes a bit too much Christmas cheer.

It's Christmastime, when we get up early, watch the children marvel at their presents under the tree, fill the den with torn wrapping paper, and thank our family for our presents even when we don't always mean it.

It's Christmastime, when we overeat at noon, doze on the couch trying to watch a boring football game, wish the children would be better behaved, hope the nieces and nephews will leave soon, and hope our spouses aren't too disappointed in the gifts we bought.

It's Christmastime, time to gather the boxes and wrapping paper for the recycle bin, time to wash the dishes, time to try to convince the children to be nice to each other on this special day, and then time to try to get them to bed.

And time for us to crash—one more Christmas in the book.

But there is another Christmas, the time we celebrate the birth of our Christian Savior, our Lord, and the Messiah. Who cares if we have co-opted the time of a pagan ritual? We know He was born. We know He lived. We know He lives still in our hearts. December twenty-fifth is as good a day as any to celebrate His birth, His life, His ministry, and even His death and resurrection.

It's Christmas. Christ is here among us. It's the time to celebrate.

So—Christmas Gift! Christmas Gift for one and all. May the world be a better place because of our Christmas Gift. May God will it so.

Memory of a Christmas Past

It was our first Christmas away from either side of our family. Carolyn and I and our infant son had moved to Philadelphia for my second year of pediatric residency. We had to adjust to living in a large city, in an Italian neighborhood where older residents spoke no English, and in the Northeast where speech patterns and food preferences were different. And we were poor. I made seventy-five dollars a month. Our rent was one-hundred-and-fifty dollars. Our families helped out.

By Christmastime, we had adjusted to life in the big city. Carolyn has a wonderful bright smile and a super outgoing personality, and she quickly made friends with our neighbors and with the corner grocer. Carolyn had introduced our little corner grocery to sweet milk, vanilla wafers, and cornmeal. He never stocked grits, despite her pleas.

We had a tree and presents—mostly for our nine-month-old son, Bill. Carolyn had something for me and I had something for her. One wintry evening on my walk to the subway, a carved ivory bracelet in a jewelry store window caught my eye. I was surprised to find that it only cost twenty dollars. That became Carolyn's Christmas present. She still wears it occasionally.

Christmas was Christmas even if it was over five-hundred miles from family. We had a tree and presents. Family sent many presents, even a whole Tennessee country ham. Carolyn carted the ham to our corner grocery to be sliced. The butcher refused. He insisted the ham was spoiled, pointing to its generous coating of mold typical of country hams. As Christmas neared, Carolyn decided we should have turkey and dressing just like home, as well. By then, the grocery had only one turkey left—a twenty-pounder. Carolyn bought it, loaded it and Bill in his little red wagon, and trundled it home.

We also had cornbread dressing—not Yankee stuffing, but real dressing. Carolyn reduced the portions from the original recipe for twelve to a recipe for two. She finally found cornmeal in a large supermarket.

Christmas came and went. We had presents, a grand Christmas meal, and best of all, a Christmas together as a family.

And our freezer was full of ham and turkey.

Christmas Parade, Country Style

It was a great way to spend a Saturday morning. I watched a Christmas parade—not a major league parade, but the small-town homefolks kind. Not only did the participants know each other, but all the spectators knew each other as well. It was in Eagleville, Tennessee, a town boasting a population of about five hundred.

We stood at the corner where two highways crossed at the only traffic light in town. The parade began right on time with the high-school band of about fifty musicians marching by the reviewing stand, which was made from a flatbed trailer.

We watched groups of men riding a variety of horses, one of which had red- and green-painted hooves. There was a group of children on ponies. Three horse-drawn buggies followed.

There were three motorcycle clubs whose roaring popping engines announced their presence. The three clubs of "hogs" were followed by a large group of adults and boys on appropriately dirty off-road bikes. There was a token female on a hog and one on a dirt bike.

A group of restored cars and trucks and several expertly restored John Deere tractors chugged by. Anyone reared in rural America could identify from a mile away the putt, putt, putt of those two-cylinder green and yellow farm machines. I expect I could still drive one of those old workhorses.

Of course, there were floats. Churches, Cub scouts, businesses, active and retired military, volunteer fire departments, and emergency medical services were represented. As usual, Santa on his float was the finale of the festivities. All floats rode on flatbed trailers pulled by pickup trucks. What the floats lacked in slick finishes was more than compensated by the enthusiasm of the children riders.

The theme, "Honoring Those Who Serve Us" was amply served by groups of active and retired soldiers, EMTs, volunteer firefighters, local politicians, law enforcement officers, businesses, the postal service, and other public servants.

The parade had no fancy floats or multiple marching bands or huge crowds or freezing weather or traffic congestion. It lasted only a half hour, and had a modest number of spectators. The weather was seasonably cold, which added to the ambience of the day. After the parade had passed, many of us adjourned to the nearby Methodist church for soup and hot chocolate.

If you are a parade fan, you might turn up your nose at this small-town, half-hour homegrown affair, but to me it was a perfect show on a perfect winter day, a welcomed part of further Christmas celebrations soon to come.

Resolutions 2010

It's January, time for those resolutions. Have you made yours yet? Do you keep them? I don't. Never have. Usually by January fifteenth, most of my resolutions lie scattered about, gasping for life. Not one survives the month.

This year, I resolved to be different. This year, I lowered the resolution bar. Why waste time on resolutions I cannot keep? Why deliberately design an activity I am guaranteed to fail?

So here they are, my resolutions for 2010:

Resolved:

To eat no purple vegetables.

Never to set an alarm clock or wear a tie except on Sunday.

To eat a piece of chocolate every day.

Never to miss a meal unless someone is in cardiopulmonary arrest.

To read the comics page every day.

Never to again try to work the New York Times crossword puzzle.

To clean my shop no more than twice a year.

To never weigh a pound less than I did in 2009.

To reply to everyone who wishes me Happy New Year with, "No thanks. I have other plans."

Never to make New Year's resolutions.

There they are, only ten. I couldn't think of twelve. I guess it only took ten to make me perfect.

Valentine Gift

There was an article on the Internet listing the ten worst Valentine's Day gifts. Since I hadn't yet bought anything for Carolyn, I read it with interest. It might prevent me from making a bad choice. Here they are, according to a Laura Gilbert who is obviously female and presumably an expert gift-receiver:

Red roses. They are predictable and clichéd, according to Laura. She suggests less common flowers, preferably in your valentine's favorite color. I gave roses once. They went over very well—but that was many years ago. We're too old for roses.

Assorted chocolates. Again, predictable and clichéd and probably there would be several pieces in the assortment that your valentine does not like. She suggests a box of one type of candy that is your valentine's favorite chocolate. I have given Carolyn chocolates before... and eaten more than my share. I often have given chocolates on February fifteenth, when the price goes down.

Jewelry in a ring-sized box. Obviously, she expects an engagement ring in that tiny box. If she is in love, the box may stir false hopes, or if unready, disappointment. Either way, you lose. The solution: nice earrings wrapped in a large box. Perhaps it would be better to skip jewelry altogether for Valentine's Day. A tiny present in a big box is a cliché if I ever saw one. I usually give jewelry for Christmas.

Sachets, candleholders, etc. Solution: Bath products. (Not a chance.)

Stuffed animal with a message of love. (Not if she is older than six.)

Racy Sleepwear: I wouldn't have the nerve to a Victoria's-Secret-type place even though I have been married to my sweetheart for over fifty-four years. She probably wouldn't wear it, anyway.

A small appliance. I would be afraid a wife or girlfriend might throw it at the giver. Carolyn has a pretty good arm.

Cologne or perfume. Chances are overwhelming she won't like the brand or the scent. Laura's solution is to buy soap or other body product with an aroma you know your valentine already has. I'll skip the fragrance idea. Carolyn is allergic to a wide variety of perfumes.

A tie. (Where did that one come from? I thought this was about a male giver and a female recipient. Carolyn doesn't wear ties.)

A gift certificate. She won't be your valentine for long if she is the recipient of this one.

This list was decidedly unhelpful. I have enough trouble with Christmas and birthdays to sweat a valentine gift. I will check a few stores and end up not buying much. Carolyn won't be disappointed. She isn't expecting much.

Independence Day Fireworks

On July fourth a few years ago, I sat on our son's back porch watching him, my son-in-law and the older grandchildren light a huge fireworks display. The show was almost as spectacular as the one in downtown Nashville. Bomb after bomb streaked into the sky, erupting with loud bangs and huge, colorful explosions. Orange, red, and blue displays burst hundreds of feet high over the lawn and the horse pasture next door. It was a spectacular show. But the most spectacular fireworks show I ever saw occurred about twenty years ago at the Brentwood Country Club.

I had joined the Brentwood Country Club, thanks to my father. He was a par golfer, one of only one or two percent of the world's amateur golfers. Needless to say, he loved the game. He gave me the money to pay my initiation fee at the country club so that he could play there when he visited us.

Since we were members, we could attend the fireworks display every year on the fourth of July—and we did. At that time fireworks at the country club bore more resemblance to backyard shoots than to corporate Brentwood or Nashville shows. Brentwood Country Club fireworks were lit manually rather than electronically; members and older children set them up and touched fuses with burning matches. Spectators sat on a gently sloping hillside oohing and aahing at each display. Shows lasted close to an hour. It was a pleasant family outing.

One show twenty years ago was a bit different. The setup and execution were similar; the results were different. Our club, like many other country clubs, had chronic financial problems. (Nobody wants to pay any more dues than are absolutely necessary.) Fortunately, our club manager located a large supply of fireworks for a ridiculously cheap price. He bought them sight unseen. The seller forgot to tell him that they had been soaked as the result of a fire in the factory the year before.

True to our minimalist fireworks tradition, our club manager carried the entire arsenal to the launch site in a pickup truck. Finally, when it became dark enough, the first bomb was lit. It flew up all of ten feet, turned north, and landed in the bed of the truck where it exploded, reminding me of the earliest NASA rocket launches. Within seconds, there were bombs bursting in air. Shrieking, zipping, whizzing, banging, booming rockets, aerial shells and florals burst above the streaking manager and his assistants, and landed all over the spectator area, bouncing off the hillside—and even a few spectators. Mothers and fathers grabbed screaming children and ran uphill away from the mayhem. We older members dodged missiles, extinguished smoldering blankets, rescued lawnchairs, and trudged up the hill away from the combat zone.

The show lasted less than ten minutes, but they were the most exciting ten minutes I ever experienced on the fourth of July.

Seasons

I like seasons. Not Minnesota seasons where summer lasts only a week or so; not Florida or Bahamas seasons where summer lasts almost the whole year. I complain about the heat of summer and the cold of winter but, to be honest, I like seasons.

Last week we returned from a short vacation in the Bahamas. Temperatures were in the mid-80s in the daylight hours and mid-70s at night. To top it off, there was a constant cooling breeze. The wonderful weather was not a surprise. Average highs from April through November range from eighty to eighty-eight. Average highs in December through March are in the mid-70s.

We spent delightful days on the beach. But what about day-to-day living there? What you get today will be what you get tomorrow. What you get tomorrow will be what you will get the next day. Perpetual summer just might be boring, only interrupted by the occasional hurricane.

Then there is Middle Tennessee. It certainly has its seasons. There is no confusing spring with summer, summer with autumn, or autumn with winter. We have no hurricanes, but we do have our seasons.

The first cold days of early winter rapidly evolve into the unrelenting onslaught of one cold day after another. Then there are the dreaded threats of snowfalls and, even worse, of ice storms. Fortunately, neither one happens with any regularity—but just often enough to cause anxiety at their threat.

February is the worst month of winter. Days in February seem colder and darker, and snow and ice seem to be more frequent. It is easy to become depressed in February. Fortunately, February lasts only twenty-eight days, and it is the month that seed catalogs come. I memorize my seed catalog now the way I did the Sears Christmas catalog when I was a young boy.

March teases. Warm days hint of spring but its warmth lives only briefly, and blustery cold seems to rule the month. There are the first warm, cloudless days of April; dangerous days, when I hurl my fragile body against the awakening earth with a vengeance. I rake dead leaves; I till and spade my vegetable gardens and flowerbeds. On many April mornings, I need to have a chain-hoist to lift me from my bed.

Spring merges with summer when there are vegetables to pick, grass to mow, weeds to pull, and shrubs to trim. Then there is the February of summer, August. June and July can be tolerated, but August must be endured. Hot day after hot day follows one after the other in relentless progression. August has the patent on sweat. August has the patent on tough weeds in the garden, on black spot on the roses, on fusarium wilt on the tomatoes and on crabgrass. Every August, I wonder if cooler weather should ever come. Must I weed and mow forever? Have I become a garden Sisyphus?

Then comes the first cool day of autumn, when an autumnal cold front transforms the hazy, muggy days of summer into a cloudless, vibrant day with a gentle, cool north breeze that clears the air and makes it sparkle like light shining off a well-cut diamond.

Fall is a time of hard labor. By then, I have become sick of gardening. The first cool days stir me to prepare my gardens for winter. I revel in the knowledge that I will not have to wield a rake or a hoe for at least five months.

Autumn is a time for football, for the World Series, for enjoying the colors of the leaves, for the anticipation of winter's nippy days. I plan for Thanksgiving and for Christmas. What is so bad about winter? Winter snows and ice are but dim pictures in my mind. I have survived many winters before. I will survive many winters to come. And if winter comes, can spring be far behind? (Apologies to Percy Shelley.)

Chapter 4, Education and Training

College, medical school, postgraduate training—eleven years of my life. I thought I was prepared for my chosen profession. Medicine had been my goal since I could remember. And then I found I was still a student, a learner forever.

Now I am retired. I don't learn as much as before. I retain a peripheral interest in medicine, but not enough to keep me from being dangerous.

The following vignettes recall some of my experiences as a permanent student.

Moonshine

My family had a farm for as long as I can remember. It was not as large as most farms in that part of the world are, but it made a good place for my father to continue his heritage as coming from farming stock. His major source of income was in business, and our farm was a minor contributor to our yearly income.

Since my father spent the majority of time in other areas, a second-in-command was essential. Mike was that person. He lived on and ran our farm for many years. He and I became close friends.

When I went off to college, my first stop upon arriving home on every holiday was at Mike's. We spent an hour or so catching up on activities on the farm and at college. During my junior year, I took organic chemistry, one of the courses required for medical school. In the laboratory a few weeks before Christmas holidays, our assignment was to make ethyl alcohol, the drinking kind. The project involved fermenting a sugar solution, distilling it, and finally, calculating the efficiency of our method.

I saved my output, about two ounces, and brought it home. The first morning home, I proudly showed Mike my product. Mike had a long history of difficulties with the authorities over his moonshining. He had been caught four times, convicted once, and served time for that offence.

Mike took my two ounces, swirled it, smelled it, and tasted a few drops. He said, "That's whiskey all right. But you didn't have to go to no fancy college to learn how to do that. I could have taught you right here on the farm and taught you how to make a whole lot more at one time, too."

Medical School

I was a freshman once again. I had been a freshman in high school, in college, and now I was a freshman in medical school. Being a freshman was becoming tiresome. Each freshman year marked a significant transition, requiring me to adapt to new surroundings.

Medical school was the biggest jump so far. I felt I had entered the academic big leagues even before the first day of classes. Of course, I needed housing—someplace close to school, someplace not too expensive, someplace close by fellow medical students. Jim, a college classmate and a friend since high school, knew several upperclassmen in one of the two medical fraternities. We attended a very casual party that served as a rush party at the fraternity house. One of the rising seniors asked Jim and me if we had rooms yet. When he learned we hadn't found one yet, he offered us the small glassed-in porch on the back of the fraternity house. It had room for two single beds and two small desks, and no heat. We took it.

I assumed that since we were living in the fraternity house, we had been accepted as members. And I guess we were—as much a member as four other freshmen who had rooms in the house.

Nobody mentioned that it was odd we had no initiation, no pin, nor were there meetings, and not a soul seemed to be an officer. I thought it strange that we owed no dues, but decided not to ask. If the fraternity wanted our dues they should ask for them. In reality, we were too busy trying to stay abreast of the mountains of work thrown at us in school to worry about the usual trappings of fraternity life. About the only evidence of fraternity was the sign in Greek letters above the front door of the house. Meetings, officers, and other fraternity stuff fell victim to the rigors of medical school for all of us.

Freshman year ran into sophomore year. Jim and I upgraded our room at the fraternity house, paid our room rent and meal costs, and stopped wondering about the lack of dues. In our third year, we moved into an apartment with two other third year students.

Some years after graduation I learned why we paid no dues. Two or three years before I entered med school, the fraternity was expelled from the national organization for non-payment of dues. No one from the national office retrieved the sign from the local fraternity. I have no idea who owned the deed to the house.

The "members" maintained the house and kept the sign. The fraternity survived quite well, unaffiliated and managed by benign anarchy.

I wonder what happened to that sign.

It Was the Worst of Days, It Was the Best of Days

Pathology was almost finished. All that was left was the final. I had survived the absolute hardest course in my second year of medical school. Some said it was the hardest two semesters of the entire four years. Few would disagree.

Dr. Shapiro, the chairman of the department of pathology, was a wounded veteran of World War II. He walked with a stiff right leg and stood at parade ground posture when addressing students. He demanded similar behavior from all students during each daily lecture and three-hour laboratory. He quizzed students throughout his lectures and labs and hurled humiliating insults at incorrect answers. Student's incorrect guesses were met by volleys of derision, sometimes tinctured by profanity. His mere presence stirred fear in his students' breasts and respect from everyone else.

I had tried to remain invisible throughout the year. I changed seats often and never asked questions. It didn't work. I received my share of Shapiro's attention. In spite of my nightly five hours of study he always dug until he exposed areas in my knowledge that were lacking.

As an experiment, the final exam in pathology was oral that year, with one faculty member quizzing a single student for an hour. The list of examiners was posted three days before exams started. We all crowded around the list to find our examiner. Of all the students and of all the faculty, my name fell on Dr. Shapiro's list. I was dead.

My medical career was over. I might as well spend my time packing. I was finished.

When I had calmed down a bit, I resolved I would not go down without a fight. I would go out kicking and screaming if I had to. And so I began my defense. I reviewed all two hundred pages of lecture notes and reread and almost memorized my seven-hundred-page pathology book. I looked over every pathology slide in several teaching collections. After three, days I felt I was as prepared as possible to meet the beast in his lair.

My turn came. I walked down the hall to his office and went in. "Don't you ever knock? You never know what might be on the other side," erupted across his desk. I gulped, went out, and knocked. Things had not begun on a good note.

For my first question, he asked, "What is the bacterial flora of the duodenum?" I was floored. I was sure that fact had never been mentioned in any lecture either in pathology or bacteriology.

I replied, "I don't know, sir."

He slammed his hand on his desk and announced, "I will not take 'I don't know' as an answer."

I knew if I guessed I was dead, but I had no option. I began to think. I knew the contents of the stomach were strongly acid, and the rapid transit of food through the duodenum might just result in a sterile environment. With trepidation, I said, "Sterile."

He said, "Of course. Everyone knows that."

The remainder of the hour was filled by questions that required me to integrate my knowledge of pathology, anatomy, and bacteriology. He even began to explain why some of my answers were off base. I began to relax a bit.

I had survived.

It was the worst of days. It was the best of days.

Influenza

We are immersed in influenza this fall. Flu to the left of us, flu to the right of us, flu ahead of us, flu behind us and rapidly catching up. We fear swine flu but keep a wary eye out for regular old-fashioned flu, too.

We agonized over whether to have the regular flu shot and whether to have the swine flu shot now that it is available to all. We may be fretting too soon and too much, but who knows? Old-fashioned flu is bad enough with high fever, severe muscle aches, terrible sore throat, wracking cough, and total prostration. A person with flu usually feels so bad he cannot lift his head from the pillow, no matter how strong his willpower.

There have been other flu epidemics with far more cases and deaths than those from swine flu so far. There was another swine flu epidemic in 1973, and there was Hong Kong flu in 1958. I have dealt with both—the first in my first year of private practice and the other in my senior year of medical school.

During my senior year of medical school, I moonlighted in an emergency room in Nashville. One evening during the height of the epidemic, I saw a lady in her thirties with typical flu. She felt terrible. I reassured her that she should recover with only symptomatic treatment.

"Won't a shot of penicillin help?" she asked.

I replied, "No. Antibiotics won't help. You should get well with fever meds and fluids. Let us see you again if you are worse in any way."

The next evening, I worked in the Vanderbilt emergency department as part of my student rotations. I walked into the exam room to see my first patient of the evening. My patient sat up and screamed, "Oh, no. Not you again!"

I quickly excused myself and asked the resident to replace me for this visit. His second opinion echoed my initial advice of the evening before.

I wonder if she ever found someone with a syringe full of penicillin.

Blood

When I was chief resident on pediatrics way back in 1962, I was responsible for all children in Vanderbilt Hospital. I supervised all the pediatric interns and residents on the pediatric wards and in the newborn nursery. It was not quite as onerous as one might guess, but I was in the hospital seven days a week, holidays included.

This was before the days of Rh immune globulin injection given to O-negative mothers during pregnancy to prevent anemia and jaundice in their offspring. Severe cases lead to deposition of bilirubin in the brain, causing significant damage. Severely affected infants were treated by exchange transfusions. Fresh O-negative blood is exchanged for the infant's damaged O-positive blood to wash out the sensitized blood and the bilirubin pigment that is the byproduct of destroyed red blood cells. Exchange transfusions were needed early in cases of severe disease.

In the course of my rounds on Christmas Day, the resident in charge of the nursery told me of one of his babies who was born with severe Rh disease. The baby needed an exchange transfusion as soon as blood was available. And there was no fresh O-negative blood in the hospital blood bank. The resident gave the problem to me. After all, that was what I was paid the princely sum of three hundred dollars a month to do—handle problems residents encountered that they couldn't solve.

I asked all the pediatric house staff in the hospital to donate blood. None were O-negative. I asked all the pediatric nurses. None spoke up. I asked all who did not know their blood type to raise their hands. I led the six responders to the blood bank, drew blood for testing from each one, and when I found the first O negative nurse I announced, "You are my volunteer donor."

The baby got his blood. The nurse got my profound thanks and the rest of the morning off. I had solved another problem, and went home for Christmas with my wife and children.

I finished my year as chief resident and went off to the NIH in Washington, D. C. for two years. When I returned to Vanderbilt, I met the director of the blood bank in the hospital hall. He looked at me intently and said, "I can't remember your name but you are O-positive."

The Dean and the Intern

Middle Tennessee is horse country. Horse stables and training rings can be found scattered throughout the countryside. I learned early in my first year of medical school that our dean fit well into the horsey set. I was told he owned a horse or two, had land enough to stable several horses, and sported a training ring near the barn. He owned the usual outfit worn for horsey meetings and contests. It was said he rarely missed riding in fox hunts during the season, but I don't know these things from personal observation.

The dean seldom spoke to students. He reserved his time for faculty and money-raising efforts. This was fine with me. The fewer contacts with those higher-ups, the better I liked it. I preferred to remain anonymous. Thus, I saw none of the following story, but several fourth year students and residents insisted it was true.

July fourth is a common day for many outdoor activities, including those involving horses. That year, there was a big horse show and cross-country race. There were flat races and at least one race over fences. Of course, horses were groomed to perfection and riders wore the traditional scarlet coat, beige riding trousers, and a black helmet despite the heat and humidity of the early July day. An ambulance stood by, ready to assist fallen riders.

According to the story, the dean was thrown during the race over fences and was suspected to have fractured an arm. He was transferred to the emergency department of Vanderbilt hospital, "his" hospital. He was seen by a freshly minted intern whose total experience was three days. (Traditionally all house staff appointments begin July first. On that day, recent graduates become interns, residents rise from intern to first-year residents, first year residents become second-year residents, and so on.)

The new intern, said to be a Harvard graduate, looked at the portly, balding, sweaty, and sunburned dean whose face was scratched, his hair mussed, and his clothes dirty and wrinkled. He carried his injured arm tucked into the front of his red jacket. The intern noted the fractured wrist on the x-ray and asked how the injury occurred.

The dean replied, "My horse threw me during a cross-country race."

The intern said, "I'll cast that arm as soon as I have time."

The dean said, "I'm the dean. I want the head of the orthopedic department to fix my arm, and I don't want to wait."

The intern stepped back, stuck his hand in the front of his white coat, and said, "And I'm Napoleon."

Nothing was ever seen of that intern again.

Algiers

News of recent riots in several Middle Eastern countries reminded me of my only experience in a Muslim country.

In 1972, I was invited by the Methodist Board of Missions to join a team of six physicians to assess the health needs of children in Algeria. The Walli (Governor) wanted to build a children's rehabilitation hospital and, to obtain the necessary foreign assistance, had to show a definite need for such a project.

The other members of our team left a few days earlier than I and were established with a missionary interpreter and an Algerian liaison officer before I arrived. I flew into Algiers (the capitol city) on the morning flight from Paris and, because my team thought I would be on the afternoon flight, no one met me. I took the lack of a reception committee with aplomb, since I knew I was to work out of the Wallyia, the Walli's office. I gathered my bag from customs, hailed a cab and, after much shouting and gesturing, set off for the Wallyia.

The cab driver deposited me in downtown Algiers, far from my ultimate destination. Downtown Algiers was a perfect copy of street scenes in the movie Casablanca. Sidewalks and streets were alive with swarthy, shabbily dressed men; some in European style clothing, some in long, loose robes, some walking, some on donkeys. Women in long, flowing robes and head covers and veils walked with eyes downcast. Street vendors shouted and displayed their wares along sidewalk edges. Streets were a chaos of cars, trucks, donkey carts, and buses, all emitting a cacophony of honks, beeps, squeals, shouts, and brays. All signs were in French or Arabic, neither of which could I read. Finally, I wandered by an international travel agency and, guessing someone there might understand English, I went in. An employee spoke a bit of English and eventually pointed me in the right direction.

Within several blocks, I came upon a small sign above a modest door that said "Wallyia". At last I had found it! I was saved!

Inside, throngs of people stood in long lines in front of battered counters, behind which bored clerks stamped forms, interviewed clients, and passed papers to the waiting people. Very soon after I entered, a firm hand grasped my elbow and propelled me up two flights of stairs to a small room containing only a desk and two chairs. After a short time, a young man in an ill-fitting, cheaply made brown business suit entered the room and began to question me. "Papers?" "Why are you in Algeria?" "Where is the rest of your party?" "In what hotel will you be registered?" "Where is your official letter of invitation?" "Do you not know Algeria does not have diplomatic relations with your country?" "Does your country know where you are?"

I replied as best I could, but, except for my passport, I had no official papers, had no invitation, did not know where my team was, and did not know the name of our hotel. He refused to believe my somewhat improbable story, and things became a bit tense.

After two hours, he left the room abruptly, returned after a time, and said, "I called the Walli's office, and you seem to be who you say you are. Your party is staying in the ________ Hotel. I have written the name and address of the hotel for a cab driver, and here is a voucher for your cab fare." I shook the man's hand, picked up my bag, and left with all deliberate speed.

By late afternoon I had registered, unpacked, strolled around the grounds, and was sitting in the dining room perusing the French language menu when the other members of the team arrived. They had met the afternoon flight, missed me, and were surprised that I was not in some Algerian jail (I was a bit surprised also.) Our missionary host quickly realized that I had entered the public entrance of the Wallyia—rather than the diplomatic entrance on the other side of the block—and had been interrogated by the secret police as a matter of routine, since I was obviously a foreigner in a place foreigners did not go. After that first day, I stayed very close to my group.

My Philadelphia Story

I was the most Southern-fried medical school graduate ever to hit the city of Philadelphia.

I grew up in a small town in rural Mississippi. I attended a small rural school and worked on our farm just enough to learn I was better suited to work with my brain rather than my muscles. When time came to select a college, my parents vetoed Mississippi universities as a rule. And so I went up east to school, to Vanderbilt, for a good education and a little polish.

After the eight years encompassing undergraduate school and medical school, I decided to go up east again to further my pediatric training. I had a good education; some of my rough rural edges had been smoothed out, but I was still very Southern in thought, actions, and speech. I looked at Johns Hopkins, Philadelphia Children's, and Boston Children's hospitals. I chose Philadelphia.

My wife, Carolyn, and nine month-old son, Bill, moved into a furnished apartment in an Italian neighborhood on the Main Line, about an hour's commute to the Children's Hospital in downtown Philadelphia.

I knew things were different up east, but I was unprepared for the degree of difference. The neighborhood grocer had never heard of sweet milk, light bread, or even vanilla wafers. The butcher refused to slice our country ham because it was moldy. Have you ever eaten scrapple? Don't. It's made of tendons, cartilage, feet, fat, and other things Southerners feed their dogs. I doubt it is even biodegradable. And they turned up their noses at country ham!

I think my fellow residents considered me to be a bit backward because I talked so slowly. They teased me about my accent and my Southern expressions such as, "I'm fixin' to do that." They had all graduated from elite Eastern schools; few had ever heard of Vanderbilt, and I detected a subtle air of condescension. It was not long before it became apparent that my education and its application equaled or excelled those of my peers.

Medical school had taught me that if one has the nurses on his side, life is immeasurably easier. In early July, a casual, "Well, bless your heart," slipped out as I thanked nurse for a favor. Her initial startled expression quickly changed to a beaming smile. "Bless your heart" was obviously a magical sentence. I used it often, and soon every nurse seemed to be in love with this Southern hayseed and could not do enough for him or his patients. Quiet suggestions and subtle warnings from experienced nurses helped me to hold my own with the best of the entire Elite East.

There are many things that are good about the South, and "bless your heart" is certainly one of them.

The Nobel Prize

Have you ever been on the centerfold of a national magazine? My wife, Carolyn and I have. Our picture appeared in Life Magazine in December 1960.

Alfred Nobel, the nineteenth-century Swedish inventor of dynamite, left most of his huge fortune to endow prizes in science, economics, and literature. Prizes are still awarded in Stockholm on December tenth every year. (The famous Peace Prize, awarded in Oslo, was begun some years after the original prizes.)

During my year's fellowship in Stockholm, I was quite flattered to receive two tickets to the white-tie awards ceremony hosted by the King and Queen of Sweden. Somewhat later I found that Swedish senior scientists, having attended dozens of these award ceremonies, routinely foisted their obligatory tickets onto their eager naïve fellows. We certainly fell into that category, but were determined not to miss a once-a-in-a-lifetime experience.

Since neither Carolyn nor I owned formalwear, we set out to rent a ball gown for her and tails for me. We had no problem finding my clothing, but nowhere in Stockholm was there a formal gown either for rent or for sale that Carolyn could wear. Swedes, as a group, are large people and very, very few Swedish women are 5'2", a hundred pounds, size six petite—and four months pregnant. Ultimately, she ordered a custom-made ball gown; expensive but worth the cost.

Carolyn felt more than a bit uncomfortable when her male tailor measured her rounding belly and her swollen bust-line. She spoke no Swedish, and he spoke no English, so we were uncertain as to exactly what style or color the gown might be. It turned out to be an elegant, black velvet two-piece evening gown that could hold its own anywhere.

We arrived at the City Hall ballroom a little early. Rather timidly, we walked through huge double doors into a gigantic room adorned with massive crystal chandeliers, large oil paintings, and sculpture. To us, neither Buckingham Palace nor Versailles could have been more opulent.

The room was filled with large tables laden with about a dozen differently shaped wine glasses and at least that many pieces of silver flatware. Plates sat on chargers, something I had never seen before. A card accompanied each place setting, and to our dismay, Carolyn was seated on one side of the room and I was seated on the other. We were two unsophisticated Americans thrown into an ultra-formal gala attended by European elite. We had not a clue as to which glass or spoon or fork we should use at which time, and now would not even have each other to lean on. Surely we would make a major social blunder and betray our plebeian American upbringings.

"Maybe we should turn around and go home," crossed my mind. But then I thought, "This is something few people get to do. We will never have this chance again. Not after our investment in clothes and a babysitter on my salary. No! We will just brazen it out." Happily, many of our tablemates were either in the same situation or were very understanding and helpful, showing us the proper glasses and forkes to use. Carolyn, a never-met-a-stranger extrovert, had a delightful evening sitting beside an Australian man who claimed he had less of a clue about glasses and silver than did she. I endured.

The Stockholm symphony played as we ate. After dessert came speeches. There were presentation speeches and acceptance speeches droning on into the night. Toward the end of the ceremony, I began to develop oratorical burnout.

The evening ended with a delightful informal mingling of all the guests in the large lobby where Carolyn and I were reunited, retrieved our coats, and walked out of the City Hall toward the subway station into gently falling snow, the first significant snowfall of winter. A perfect ending to our once-in-a-lifetime Nobel experience.

Addendum:

Our picture and those of the Nobel Laureates, the King and Queen of Sweden and four-hundred-and-ninety-eight other guests appeared on the centerfold of Life Magazine the next week. My mother-in-law saved the issue for us, but I was never able to identify either Carolyn or myself, even using a magnifying glass. But indeed, we were there.

Sjukvård

Toward the end of my post-graduate medical training, a fellowship to study immunochemistry in Stockholm, Sweden just fell into my lap. I had not even applied for it, but there it was, a gift arranged by my Vanderbilt professor of pediatrics. Since my career goal at that time was to become a research scientist in infectious diseases and their immune responses, the offer of a year's study in laboratories that led the world in the chemistry of the immune system was a gift from heaven and something that could not be turned down. I jumped at the offer like a bass striking a crayfish. Carolyn had her doubts and second thoughts about living a year in Stockholm with her two children— me and our one-year old son—but I didn't.

Six months before departure, I began to study Swedish. I bought a course that combined a written text and a series of 33 RPM records. I spent hours learning basic Swedish, and by the time we arrived, could manage a very simple conversation—sort of.

A year's residence, listening to Swedish radio, dealing with Swedish shop clerks and public transit workers, and watching American movies with Swedish subtitles improved my Swedish considerably. I could ask directions and understand replies; I could order a meal; I could shop at the fish store, the bakery, the vegetable store, the butcher shop, and could tell the barber how I wanted my hair to be cut. I was comfortable in Swedish, but not fluent. On the other hand, Carolyn only knew three phrases in Swedish: eighty Swedish cents for subway fare to our station, a common, cheap and tasty crappie-like fish, and how to tell the barber to cut our son's hair short.

I learned that I should never leave our apartment without a jacket and tie, even to go fishing; I could identify American tourists by their dress and by their body language. I learned to eat raw herring, reindeer, poached fish, I ate boiled potatoes almost every day and learned to peal my potatoes on my plate using my knife and fork the way the Swedes do. I never could eat raw ground meat mixed with beets, onion, and capers, but I noticed that many Swedes also asked to have their beef cooked.

By spring, Carolyn was once again massively pregnant. (She began to show about three days after conception.) She craved steak and a green salad, but the only beef in Sweden came from post-menopausal dairy cows and could only be cut by a recently-sharpened chainsaw. Fresh vegetables were kept at night in vaults they shared with jewelry stores, and there was not a leaf of lettuce in all of Stockholm.

For Carolyn's birthday, early in her ninth month of pregnancy, we hired a babysitter and dined at a moderately expensive restaurant. Since she could not read or speak Swedish, I ordered. There were no lettuce salads on the menu, but horse-meat steaks were featured. It was the best beef we had all year. Carolyn only found out later.

We had our second child, a girl, three weeks before we were to sail for home. It was a frantic time of caring for a newborn baby, registering her birth at the United States Embassy, packing a year's worth of stuff, arranging ship passage for ourselves and our car, and planning for the three-hundred-and-fifty-mile drive from Stockholm to Gothenburg.

Carolyn had not fully recovered from her delivery and still could not sit comfortably. As an ever-loving husband, but up to now, a rather marginal provider, I set out to buy a rubber ring to ease her cross-country ride.

"Rubber ring" was not in my English-Swedish dictionary so I had to describe it. I went from shop to shop to shop all afternoon speaking in Swedish… to a first clerk, then to a second clerk, and finally to a manager or owner. "No, we do not carry such an item," echoed in my ears all afternoon. Each shop politely referred me to another possible provider until I finally found the ring in a "Sjukvård", a store that sold rubber goods—a contraceptive shop.

The Consultant

My morning's mail contained a request for donations to help establish a two-million dollar endowment for the new Eugene Braunwald Clinical Investigator Award in memory of Dr. Braunwald. The letter mentioned his contributions to our knowledge of heart failure, coronary artery disease, and their treatment among other significant discoveries. He is considered to be one of the most distinguished cardiologists of our time. I had one brief encounter with Dr. Braunwald.

I met Dr. Braunwald during my postgraduate training at the National Institute of Allergy and Infectious diseases. I was in my first of two years studying viral illnesses from the clinical perspective as well as in the laboratory. Part of my duties involved care for a number of inpatients with a variety of infectious or autoimmune diseases. One of my patients was a young, previously healthy man who had been admitted to the cardiology institute because of severe, painful, angina-like chest pain. Studies revealed evidence of pericarditis, an inflammation of the heart muscle and of the pericardium, the sack surrounding the heart. In addition to pain, signs of fluid often accompany the illness. Since the condition is almost always caused by a virus, the cardiologists requested an infectious diseases consultation. It was my turn to do consults and so I went.

My exam revealed a most significant finding—an abnormal heart sound, a rub. A rub is exactly what the name implies—a rasping sound similar to the sound of sandpaper on wood or a rasp shaping wood. None of the cardiologists had made note of such a sound, but it was clearly there when I examined him. I had no doubt. I mentioned the rub in my note and suggested they obtain specimens for me to test for one of the many viruses that can cause pericarditis.

My boss, the head of the clinical infectious diseases division, called me the next day. He said, "Dr. Eugene Braunwald is visiting the cardiac institute and would like to see your patient with pericarditis. We have arranged for a clinical conference tomorrow and you will present the patient to Dr. Braunwald."

I had finished medical school and had three years of postgraduate training and one year's fellowship at that time, so I was no novice. But to present a patient to such a distinguished man in front of the chiefs of cardiology and infectious diseases, all their fellows and a few other important people did engender a bit of anxiety, enough to ensure that I would be well-prepared.

Dr. Braunwald was about sixty or so, gray haired, and a bit overweight. He wore a wrinkled dull brown suit and seem to have a twinkle in his eyes and a half-smile on his lips—a benign grandfatherly old man. I presented my patient's history and my physical findings. I was especially thorough in my description of his rub. Dr. Braunwald pulled out his stethoscope and spent a remarkably long time listening to my patient's heart. He listened while the patient was flat on his back, when the patient lay on his right side, when he lay on his left side, and even when he sat up and leaned forward.

Finally, Dr. Braunwald pointed to a spot on the patient's left chest between the sternum and left nipple and announced, "Right there sounds like where a rub was yesterday."

I also listened. Not a smidgen of rub was present. Dr. Braunwald proceeded to expound on the symptom of pericarditis and how rubs can be frustratingly evanescent. The world-famous cardiologist had bailed out the lowly trainee.

I think I will make a small donation to that fund.

The Kennedy Assassination

What were you doing on November 22, 1963—the day an assistant press secretary announced, "President John F. Kennedy died at approximately one o'clock Central Standard Time today, here in Dallas"?

I walked into my research lab in the National Institutes of Health that day and saw my assistant, a tall, heavily built, balding black man sitting by the window, crying. He sobbed, "President Kennedy has been killed!" I don't remember much of the rest of the day but I left at my accustomed time in the late afternoon.

Carolyn had spent the afternoon watching TV, sitting with her foot beneath her, folding diapers and watching the unfolding drama of the assassination while the older children played and our baby napped. The day was filled with medical reports, the swearing-in of Vice President Lyndon Johnson, and even speculation about a possible political coup. When she stood, her numb ankle turned beneath her, resulting in an immediate painful baseball-size swelling. I insisted we go to the National Naval Medical Center where we usually received our medical care. Little did we know that President Kennedy's body was to be taken there.

At the hospital, we encountered a six-foot-four Marine holding a rifle with a fixed bayonet guarding the emergency entrance. After some persuasion, he allowed us into to the Emergency Department, where Carolyn was x-rayed, given crutches, and dismissed. Then came a problem. The same Marine refused to let us leave! He listened to our pleas with world-class deafened ears—and at six-four with a rifle and bayonet, threats and pleas would have bounced off him like BBs off a tank.

We were herded into a small, windowless room off the main hospital entrance and forced to remain there, cut off from the outside world. We had no access to TV or a telephone. Fortunately, a very responsible teenager was caring for our children. Dozens of arrogant, aggressive newsmen milled about in the room and discussed rumors of a possible military coup. Armed Marines were everywhere. No one knew anything. Some of them began to listen for sounds of distant gunfire. Finally, we saw grim-faced generals and admirals parade by, not twenty feet away. They were followed by Bobby and Ethyl Kennedy, Ted and Joan Kennedy, Eunice and Sergent Shriver, and then Jackie, still in her pink, blood-spattered suit and pillbox hat. Once they had passed, we were allowed to leave.

We hobbled home at about ten o'clock, tired, hungry, and shaken. We had lived through another of those rare days like Pearl Harbor or the death of President Franklin Roosevelt that was etched clearly in our memories forever.

Adventures in the Federal Prison System

I have been in most of the federal correctional facilities in the Southeast.

I spent most of two years at the National Institutes of Health doing research into the virology of the common cold. Before you dismiss this effort as another federal waste of money, be aware that the common cold is responsible for a major loss of work time, a huge slice of the over-the-counter drug cost, and significant numbers of doctor visits.

As part of our research effort, we inoculated healthy volunteers with cold viruses and studied their clinical and immunologic responses to the infection. Our volunteers came from inmates of the federal prison system. As part of my duties, I visited most of the minimum-security facilities in the Southeast to recruit our subjects.

"Minimum security" meant just that. Guards and fences were minimal. The facility at Pensacola had no fences at all. It was built in the middle of a huge, trackless area containing only scrub pine, palmettos, and snakes. I asked the superintendent if escapes were prevalent.

He replied, "We had two inmates walk off a couple of years ago. They came back after two days and begged us to take them back."

The federal prison system has an extensive educational program. Inmates can earn their GEDs or learn a variety of skills useful for future employment once they are released. I noticed a substantial number of inmates incarcerated for moonshining were taking courses in welding. A convicted counterfeiter was in a course on calligraphy.

Chosen inmates spent one month in the National Institutes of Health clinical facility while we followed their clinical and immunologic responses to infections with cold viruses. They ate good food and had extensive recreational opportunities, including a visit to a major league baseball game in the summertime.

We also arranged for them to have minor surgical procedures during their stay. Tattoo removal was quite popular until stopped by the prison system. We were removing identifying marks.

Rarely did an inmate escape or misbehave. Any trouble resulted in their summarily being transferred to the District of Columbia Federal Jail, a facility widely known and feared throughout the federal prison population.

Once, after an inmate walked off and was promptly recaptured, we endured a lecture by a federal marshal on security. He outlined procedures we were to use in holding a runaway until the marshals arrived.

Our boss commented after the lecture, "Thank you for your information. If I happen to see one of our subjects on the street I will advise him to return to the NIH promptly."

Leprosy

A story in a recent sermon in my church that mentioned leprosy stimulated memories of my experience with this disease.

Part of my responsibilities at the National Institutes of Health included clinical care for three young men infected with the leprosy bacillus. The three were part of a study of new drugs to treat this chronic infection. My responsibilities included clinical evaluation of the progression or, as was hoped, the regression of the infection.

Do not classify me as an infectious disease hero for my efforts. Contrary to one's impression from the Bible, the disease is minimally contagious and usually is transmitted only by close contact over a prolonged time. It is most typically transmitted only to family members in poor, primitive circumstances. Transmission in environments with ordinary hygiene of modern life occurs, rarely if at all.

Even so, our three lepers caused considerable fear among non-medical people. This was not all bad. While I was at the NIH, it was not uncommon for members of Congress and other politicians high on the influence scale to call requesting a hospital stay for their spouses for exhaustion, fatigue, nervousness, or other equally vague symptoms. Institute chiefs were loath to deny such requests from high-ranking politicians even though almost all of these admissions were more social than medical. Every clinical institute but ours was affected.

Whenever our chief received such a call, he is said to have replied like this: "Senator, we would be happy to admit your spouse for tests. But I would like to warn you that we have three lepers on our wards."

During my two years at the NIH we never had one social admission.

It was during my second year at the NIH, when I had recovered from the awe of working in the premier medical research facility in the nation, that I made a request. I knew that there was a facility caring for leprosy in Carvel, Louisiana. It was funded by the federal government and staffed by physicians in the Public Health Service. They received extra pay for hazardous duty, though everyone knew there were few if any hazards connected with their duties.

I thought that since I took care of lepers, maybe I deserved hazardous duty pay, as well. Mostly tongue-in-cheek, I composed a letter requesting hazardous duty pay. My request never left my boss's desk except to return to me stamped "denied."

Yellow Berets

Last year's Veteran's Day activities stirred memories of my service in my country's defense.

I was too young to serve in World War II. My age fit perfectly for the Selective Service System to grab me up in its gigantic arms to send me to Korea. I was seventeen when the shooting started, and twenty when an armistice was signed. Fortunately, the word "selective" was included in the title of the system designed to draft an army. Deferments were easy to obtain then. All a young man needed to do was to stay in some kind of school and make a C average.

Making a C average was a piece of cake for me. I was a pre-med student and worked hard to make the good grades necessary to qualify for medical school. Grades bought me my deferment as an incidental benefit. I did take ROTC for two years and learned how to salute, to march, and to wear a uniform. Little did I know that ROTC was to be the total extent of my exposure to the niceties of military life. Cleaning and shooting a rifle were old hats to me, since I had my own .22 caliber rifle. I had hunted birds and rabbits with a borrowed shotgun.

Medical school and internship meant automatic deferment. I signed into another plan that guaranteed my further deferment through my post-medical school training. In 1962, after medical school and four years of post-medical training, I was inducted into the military services at age twenty-nine.

I was fortunate to have been assigned the rank of Lieutenant Commander in the Coast Guard and ordered to do research in my former teacher's laboratories at the National Institutes of Health. There were no uniforms, no saluting, and no formations at the NIH. We were told just to work hard, draw our officer's pay, and discharge our military obligations.

I had one of the cushiest jobs in the entire uniformed services of the United States Government, and I didn't even have a uniform. The guys in the real navy called us "Yellow Berets."

But things have a way of changing.

In October 1962 came the Cuban missile crisis. The Soviet Union began to install missiles in Cuba that were capable of reaching most of the United States with nuclear warheads. The escalating crisis resulted in my unit of twelve thoroughly non-military scientists receiving orders to take tropical illness vaccines and remain on twelve-hour alert to ship out. Nobody would tell us where we were to go or what we would do when we got there, wherever "there" was. I wondered what chaos might ensue when this crew of civilian scientists arrived at some military facility looking for our assignment.

The crisis died. We continued our research.

Nobody called us Yellow Berets anymore.

What to Do, What to Do?

I fulfilled my military obligation by doing research at the National Institutes of Health just outside of Washington, D.C. Since I had one of the cushiest jobs in the whole United States military, my friends in the Naval Medical Center across the street called me a "Yellow Beret". Few sailors called us that after the Cuban Missile Crisis in 1962, when my unit was placed on twelve-hour alert and received yellow fever, cholera, and typhoid fever vaccines.

During the crisis, airwaves resounded with warnings of a likely nuclear attack on the Washington, D.C. area if shooting started. Civil Defense officials selected public fallout shelters, but our shelter was not stocked—Civil Defense had run out of proper forms. Even though we lived at the edge of the zone of total destruction, I made a makeshift fallout shelter by running a garden hose from our water heater to our 10x15 foot basement pantry. At least we had something, no matter that it was poor protection at best.

We had a two-year-old and a four-year-old and my wife, Carolyn, was expecting to deliver our third child any day. Our best friends, Joan and Dewey, had three preschool children. Carolyn and Joan each kept one hundred dollars in cash and made sure that one of them had a car with a full tank of gas at home every day.

Our fears rose when we learned that US warships were steaming toward a Soviet ship loaded with long-range missiles bound for Cuba. To stop the ship and seize the missiles would be an act of war, and might likely result in a Soviet nuclear missile strike. Washington, D.C. would surely be target number one.

What to do? What to do? Carolyn and Joan discussed their options.

If missiles flew, neither Dewey nor I, if we survived, could go home. We would be on our way to a field hospital somewhere.

The official Washington evacuation plan called for people living in our area to go northwest past Fort Dietrich, Maryland, the only army biological warfare facility in the country. Evacuation did not seem to be a viable option.

Carolyn and Joan agreed that, if they survived the blast, four weeks in that small room, our "fallout shelter," with five young children was not survivable.

What to do? What to do? They knew what to do. They put the children in the navy daycare center for the day, pocketed their one hundred dollars and went shopping.

Chapter Five, Family

This section is unorganized and spans subjects from children to grandchildren to pets to retirement.

Over the Hill and Through the Woods to Grandmother's House

Twice a year, our Georgia connection comes to town. Our older daughter, her husband, and their four children live near Athens, Georgia, and visit us at Christmastime and in midsummer. They left for home three hours ago.

Since cousins like to be together, our four Middle-Tennessee grandchildren spent most of the ten days at our house as well, forming an ever-moving, ever-eating mélange of adolescents and pre-adolescents—four boys and four girls who range in age from five to seventeen. The Georgia clan and the two of us filled our four bedrooms—and when cousins slept over, sleeping bags covered every floor.

Do you remember how much food adolescents consume? Elephants put away two hundred pounds of food a day, an amount easily matched by our four adolescent grandsons and approached by our two older granddaughters. Where the calories go is a mystery. Not one grandchild has an ounce of excess fat. One-hundred-forty cans of soft drinks, ten gallons of lemonade, three gallons of milk, one-and-a-half gallons of ice cream, and seventy-two Popsicles disappeared in ten days. A turkey breast, a pot roast, half a ham, a three-pound meatloaf, six pounds of barbeque, six pounds of shrimp, seven large pizzas, and fifteen pounds of catfish are missing. We cooked three pounds of dried white beans from the grocery, four quarts of green beans, four quarts of peas, and forty ears of corn from the garden. Homegrown tomatoes, cucumbers, squash and blackberries rounded out their diet.

Lucky Charms and Pop-Tarts suddenly appeared on the breakfast menu. Breakfasts ran from eight to eleven, lunches from eleven to three and dinners from five to eight. Of course, there were also snacks in between.

Ten to fifteen people ate most meals with us, but last night we fed twenty-two as nieces, nephews, great-nieces, great-nephews, boyfriends and girlfriends swelled the guest list. Carolyn never left the kitchen for ten days. I spent most of my time at the grocery store. I haven't seen the statistics yet but I expect to see an upward blip in the national retail sales figures for July.

Six bicycles of various sizes, two tricycles, a motorized toy Jeep, a croquet court and a shuffleboard court provided outside diversions but the most popular activity was Hide and Seek played at night with "it" armed with a flashlight. They call it "German Spotlight" for reasons that escape me. Other entertainment included golf for the boys, horseback riding for the girls, and movies and Nashville Shores for them all.

Our house has a computer, four television sets, three bathrooms, and a washer and a dryer. All were in continuous use throughout the entire ten-day visit. The upstairs den seemed always to hold several grandchildren—one on the computer, some watching TV, some playing board games, and all eating. Now that we are alone, we are considering just raking out the den and hosing it down.

After teary-eyed farewells were over, I watched the final round of the British Open golf tournament and reclaimed my computer. These simple pleasures were somehow less satisfying than I had anticipated, and the house seemed far too quiet. But we will be able to see everyone again in six short months, and Carolyn is reasonably sure she can restore our house to its pre-visit state by then.

Retirement

At the time of this writing I have been creatively unemployed for more than seven years, drawing my Social Security pension (partially financed by my hard-working children) and saying to myself each morning, "What fun thing can I do today?"

I have had only one bad day in retirement; I saw my dentist and my tax bill on the same day.

For several weeks after I had retired, I toyed with the idea of "alternative transportation". A motorcycle would be dangerous, impractical, and totally unnecessary—an irresistible combination. But there was a better way, a safer way to learn to ride a motorized bicycle, a cheaper way to ride a motorized bicycle. I needed a moped!

A tour through the yellow pages revealed only one dealership with a moped for sale. It was located in a neighborhood of tenements, bars, discount stores, and pawnshops. No matter. I needed a moped. I drove my truck (bought a year before in anticipation of retirement) to the motorcycle store, and as I dismounted, met a customer walking out. He was about six-feet-two, wore faded blue jeans that had more holes than intact cloth, a black biker's tee-shirt, large swastikas tattooed on each arm, a three-day beard, a long, dirty blond pony-tail, and wore an American flag do-rag.

Inside were four men who fit a similar profile. All were smoking—tobacco, I think. The owner was a clone of Danny Devito, only shorter, fatter, and balder. The mechanic was as tall, lean, and pale as a cadaver, reminding me of a character in the TV show "The Addams Family". He had a jet-black ponytail and carried a scar on the left side of his face from his hairline to his chin—but he was a nice guy. A young salesman wore a dirty tee-shirt, a dirty blond ponytail, Bermuda shorts, and a semi-automatic pistol tucked into his belt.

I was afraid not to buy the moped.

Finding a Church

Our family moved to the Brentwood/Oak Hill area in 1964, forty-seven years ago. The first thing we did after unpacking was to look for a church.

I set out with our older two children (ages three and five years) in our Volkswagen Beetle in search of a church on the first Saturday in our new home. Carolyn stayed home with our youngest, a one-year-old. We drove to the Crievewood United Methodist Church first. At that time, it was merely a tarred-over basement that served as Sunday School and Sanctuary. We had come from a church just like that in Maryland, and I turned the Crievewood church down out of hand. I wanted a real church instead of a make-do church. I was tired of efforts to raise money for a building, as well.

I headed to Brentwood, right down the road. Surely a town the size of Brentwood would have a Methodist church. I grew up in a town of one thousand, and it had six churches. Brentwood should be the same. And there, on the corner of Church Street and Franklin Road in downtown Brentwood stood this little, brick, Gothic-style Methodist Church. We pulled into the parking lot, and the children and I went in. As soon as we entered, we met the sexton, Stokes. He quickly asked about our family and gave us a tour of the church, making sure to point out the nursery and the Sunday School classrooms for three-year-olds, five-year-olds, and young married couples.

He also took us to the sanctuary. I loved the warm, inviting ambience of the walnut-covered vaulted ceiling and wainscoting. Light from the arched stained-glass windows added to the overall feeling of peace and reverence.

When we arrived home, I told Carolyn, "I think I have found us a new church. It's built in a beautiful old Gothic style, and if everyone is as welcoming as the sexton, we should fit right in. Besides, the cornerstone says it was founded in 1852, so it's probably paid for."

Within two years, there was talk of how badly we had outgrown our little church, formation of a building fund, and a march down Franklin Road to a new campus. Three major additions have resulted in a one-hundred-and-eighty-five-thousand square-foot facility housing a congregation of about seven-thousand-and-five-hundred.

The building will be paid off soon.

Quinqs

The year 2008 was something special. I was inducted into the Vanderbilt Medical School as a Quinq—a graduate of fifty years ago.

Seventeen of the forty-six graduates of the class of 1958 were honored with medallions, certificates, fancy pens, and fancy notepaper. Fifteen classmates had died—almost forty percent, a high death rate it seems to me. But doctors seem to do that, to be "ridden hard and put up wet." We don't seem to last long, but we have a wonderful ride getting there.

Breakfast on Friday was held to recognize our class. I looked around the room. There were several I would not have recognized, and others I barely did. In contrast to ten years ago, the few trophy wives had aged into elegant ladies. (Carolyn wanted to outlaw trophy wives at reunions.)

All the men seemed to be a bit stooped, a bit potbellied, and what hair they had left was gray. Such are the ravages of time. But we were here; we were upright; we were warm; we were pink; most of us were mobile; most of us knew where we were.

The breakfast festivities ended at two p.m. to reconvene at a dinner dance that evening. Most of us left at about ten that evening. I remember in college and medical school when parties barely started by ten. But Carolyn and I and our houseguests, a classmate and his wife of fifty years (like us), drove home only to relive old memories of fifty years ago until one a.m.

Saturday began a new day. We and our houseguests enjoyed a delightful brunch with my two other closest medical school friends and their wives before the football game that afternoon. We spent three delightful hours reminiscing once again. We four guys were the very closest friends that I had ever experienced. We dissected a cadaver together; we roomed together beginning with our freshman year; we were in each other's weddings; we partied together. We called ourselves "the four horsemen", as trite as it was. Our guests and we were pleased we had missed the debacle at Dudley field.

Saturday night brought our class party, an elegant dinner dance at the Belle Meade Country Club. We eight classmates sat together once again—but not for a final time if we are lucky.

We had four parties over two days, each one an elegant happening, each one filled with nostalgia, each one an unforgettable meeting, each one a memorable experience. Five years from now, our backs will have become more stooped, our hair will have thinned even more, and our short-term memories will have diminished, but the love among the four horsemen will remain as strong as ever.

Evergreen

Many years ago when our children were two, four, and six, Carolyn joined some of her friends for a well-deserved three-day weekend sabbatical at Red Boiling Springs. I was left with the children for the long weekend.

At Friday breakfast, the children and I discussed plans for the weekend. The two older ones wanted to build a treehouse. Since Mother was out of town, she was in no position to hear about our plans, and, of course, could not veto the whole project.

We selected a large tulip maple tree in the backyard to hold our treehouse and piled into my Volkswagen Bug for a trip to the lumber yard. We returned home with a generous supply of lumber tied to the rooftop luggage rack and set to work.

I persuaded the children to place the treehouse only about fifteen feet high and to limit the house to a platform with a strong rail around it for safety. I built a ladder into the design, as well.

Once we had finished construction, the children insisted we paint the treehouse. We selected a can of forest-green enamel and four cheap brushes at the hardware store. As soon as we had begun to paint, neighborhood children began to gather. Eventually, we had a large group of friends from the neighborhood clamoring to help.

And so, I let them. Soon paint, accidently at first and intentionally later, began to find its way onto children's bodies. By the time we had finished, we had a green treehouse, green handprints in the refrigerator, on the storm door, and on most of my tools. The neighborhood was overrun with green children—hardly a restful color, under the circumstances.

Reckoning came all too soon. Carolyn returned, and the neighborhood children went home. It seemed every mother in the neighborhood, including Carolyn, felt it necessary to explain to me the principles of childcare—including avoiding forest-green paint. Eventually the paint was cleaned off the refrigerator, and, in time, wore off the evergreen children.

Mother Goose

Mother Goose is not a myth. She did exist, though the facts of her life are in some dispute. One version of her life places her in Boston, England, while another account places her in Boston, Massachusetts. Since I have seen her gravestone and that of her son-in-law, Thomas Fleet, in Boston, Massachusetts, I feel the following account, taken from the April 1059 Reader's Digest, is most probably true.

"There was an old woman who lived in a shoe, who had so many children she didn't know what to do." Almost everybody is brought up on Mother Goose, but few know that the old lady was a Bostonian. In 1660, the Gooses owned nearly half of Boston. There were ten little Gooses, and their father, Isaac, took Elizabeth Foster for his second wife, who had ten children of her own and became the immortal Mother Goose.

"After Isaac died, she went to live with her eldest daughter, who had married Thomas Fleet, a printer who lived in Pudding Lane, now Devonshire Street. The Fleets had a whole house full of children, and Mother Goose used to sing songs and ditties all day long. Other children swarmed to Pudding Lane to sit on the stoop and hear her. Finally, her son-in-law gathered her jingles together and printed them, never realizing that he had a bestseller. Neither did Mother Goose, who lived to be a hundred, and died mumbling, "Humpty Dumpty sat on a wall."

Yes, Mother Goose did indeed exist—and, though not genetically related to me, she is still family. The American

Fleet name can be traced back to 1621, when Henry landed at Jamestown, Virginia. Fleets spread from Virginia to New England, to Tennessee, to Texas, to Colorado, to California, to Oklahoma, and to Mississippi.

Though I cannot trace my lineage to Mother Goose, I'm sure she fits into our family tree somewhere.

Our youngest daughter attended middle school at Harpeth Academy in Franklin. Harpeth Academy's sixth grade contained several snooty, haughty, pre-adolescent girls. They constantly bragged about their fathers' statuses as a doctor, a lawyer, and a mayor, and to top it off, their mothers' memberships in the DAR.

Poor Patricia. She had nothing to brag about. Carolyn dug out the Reader's Digest article for her to read in class. Nobody bragged about family after that.

Et Tu, Brute?

The single positive thing about February is that it lasts only twenty-eight days. Four years ago, on the first Tuesday in February, I arose at seven-fifteen, brushed my teeth, drank a cup of super-strong coffee to get my heart started, read the A-section of the paper, and left shortly before eight o'clock for my Tuesday breakfast club meeting.

I belong to the "Burger Boys Breakfast Club", which now meets at Dimple's Deli. It is an ideal organization. There are no dues, no attendance requirements, no officers, and no projects. Just twenty-five old guys who meet once a week and take over the deli at breakfast-time.

I left the deli into slate-gray skies and spitting snow. I had no woodworking projects to do, it was too cold to fish, and Carolyn had a lunch date with friends. I had no other plans for the day, but I was right on schedule. I filled the morning with a trip to the grocery and by reading my book of the week.

At noon came the mail. Included was the final piece of data to allow me to complete my income tax forms. After a hotdog and a salad, I began to complete them. I finished at three-thirty, totally drained. I returned to my easy chair, too tired to pick up my book and turned on the TV. A channel-surf landed me on "Turner Classic Movies". I watched Marlon Brando in Act Three, Scene Two of Shakespeare's Julius Caesar, where Mark Antony mourns Caesar's death.

The speech is laced with wonderful lines.

"Friends, Romans and Countrymen; lend me your ears! Wounds like dumb mouths do open their ruby lips to beg the voice and utterance of my tongue; I came to bury Caesar not praise him; The evil that men do lives after them, the good is often interred with their bones; This was the most unkindest cut of all."

And throughout the two-page speech, Shakespeare weaves the accusatory thread, "for they were honorable men." Shakespeare and Brando saved a bummer afternoon.

Even after four hundred years, Shakespeare can stir emotions. I realized again what a puny thing my writing is. Going one-on-one with Michael Jordan, Pete Sampras, or Tiger Woods would be no picnic either, but I think I might look better against them than I would look against Old Will.

Guitar Man

I was a guitar player until about thirty years ago. Guitar players in Nashville are not at all rare. In fact, you can find one on almost every streetcorner in downtown Nashville.

My guitar playing took a totally different path than did almost all of Nashville's aspiring string musicians. I took up the guitar when I was mature—at least physically. I had a paying job, however modest, and was happily married with three healthy, lively children.

I was comfortably ensconced in my niche as a fulltime researcher and teacher in the department of pediatrics in the Vanderbilt School of Medicine. Although I worked long hours at the school, I still had some time for outside interests—one of which was music.

An ad stating the Metro-Nashville Public school system's schedule for nighttime adult education classes appeared in our newspaper in early fall. There was a class in guitar for beginners at Overton High School, only three blocks from my house.

Playing a guitar makes a person the center of attraction in any group. Playing a guitar could make me a star, if only among my closest friends. I signed up. Why not? It was free—except that I needed a guitar. A trip to a music store yielded me a decent, cheap instrument, good enough for a beginner.

The class was not exactly free. We needed a book, which was, surprisingly enough, written by our teacher.

But it was a good book, a helpful book, and one that would really help me learn to play the guitar.

I attended each weekly class faithfully. I practiced at least an hour every night. I studied music theory and chord progression and began to appreciate the complexities and the beauty of music. I began to love it.

I took an intermediate class, continued to practice, and began to branch out to more advanced endeavors. Soon, I learned to play two parts on my guitar at the same time. I could play two parts of "Fera Jaca" simultaneously. Then came "Dueling Banjos." I learned to play both of the slower first parts simultaneously. I began to learn Chet Adkins' style. I began to feel almost qualified for the Grand Ole Opry.

Then I saw an ad on the bulletin board in our grocery store reading, "Classical guitar lessons, beginners only."

I thought, "I would really like to play classical guitar. Here's my chance to become another Andres Segovia." I called the number on the ad. "I don't know if I am a beginner or not," I said. "I can play melody and chords and two parts of music at the same time."

"Come play for me and we will see."

And so, I did. When I finished he said, "You are a beginner—no question about that."

A Love Letter

My esteemed editor asked me to write something about my love affair with my wife. Though I loved her from our first meeting, I found it difficult to write about our fifty-three years together. Instead, I moved back two generations.

We found this letter after my grandmother died. It was written about one year after her first husband died.

Wintersville, Mo.

Aug. 31, 1903

Mrs. Dora Callahan,

Kind Friend, will try to write you a few lines. You will no doubt be surprised in receiving this but I hope not offended. What I wanted to ask you is that I might have the pleasure of your company some Sunday evening.

I have been wanting to ask you for this privilege ever since last winter but was afraid to. I thought that perhaps you didn't want to keep company with anyone. I hear that you are keeping company with another fellow and you needn't think that I am just trying to cut him out just for the name of it for it isn't as I haven't a thing against him.

Now if you don't want to keep company with more than one fellow and would rather go with him than me say so and I will take my medicine like a man and we will be as good friends as in the past.

If your answer is yes, can you name a day when and where you will be at that time. If your answer to this letter is no, please don't tell any more people than necessary not that I am ashamed of writing this as I would deem it an honor but you know some people don't have any mercy on a person's feelings especially before a crowd. If your answer should be no but I hope not for that is nearly as bad a word as never. Please return this in your letter ....(unreadable)

Please answer this soon as you can conveniently.

Please excuse all mistakes and blunders.

Hoping for a favorable reply I remain,

(s)Harper P. Vance

They married in 1904. Harper's great grandfather was Samuel Harper, who came to America from Scotland in 1754 and settled along the Potomac River at what is now known as Harper's Ferry, Virginia, a place of some importance in Civil War history.

I find it difficult to improve upon this love letter.

My Granddog, Sadie

She entered my life fourteen years ago, a little big-pawed puppy as black as the inside of a coal mine. She was a cute little thing, snuffling about on her panther paws in the mudroom where she was confined. She ate and sniffed and drooled and licked everything within reach. She especially liked human company. She had the makings of an ideal pet for my five-year-old grandsons. They named her, Sadie.

Nobody's perfect, not even dogs; not even purebred cute little black Labrador puppy dogs. Puppies like to chew. Labradors are known for their propensity to chew. Sadie developed into a magna cum laude chewer. She began small, destroying all her chew toys. She progressed to her plastic dog dishes, then an assortment of garden shoes. Soon she tackled greater challenges. She ate the tires off the twins' plastic ride-in Jeep as a preliminary exercise preceding bigger challenges.

She ate a hole through the drywall sheeting separating the garage from the storeroom where she slept. As a finale, she ate the wiring out of the parking lights of my daughter-in-law's van.

Adulthood brought forth the dog her puppy conformation had promised. She became a sleek black collection of muscle and bones, eager to behave herself and to obey her master's commands. Her mild manner was only challenged when yappy little dogs pushed her too far.

Now poor Sadie is fourteen years old. She is inflicted with a myriad of geriatric ills. She is deaf, can hear only loud shouts and clapping; she had a stiff arthritic rear leg; she can no longer run without becoming short of breath; she can no longer climb steps. Her vision is suspect.

But Sadie remains a lovable, loving old senior citizen. She reminds me of me.

Moses

My wife, Carolyn found him at a gas station—a lost or abandoned, injured, starving six-month-old puppy. When our veterinarian released him three days later, Carolyn and our daughter, Tricia, took him to an animal shelter. After learning that the shelter did not have a safe place for a not-yet-well puppy, Carolyn looked down into Tricia's two teary brown eyes. "Put the dumb dog in the car. We're taking him home!" she snapped.

Moses had adopted us.

Moses was a mixed breed of average size, somewhat shorter and less muscular than a German Shepherd. He had a shepherd's muzzle and a hound's ears and walked with turned-in, "cow-hocked" hind legs. He was white with large black spots and resembled my childhood dog, Moses (the reason for his name).

Although he was far from an imposing specimen of doghood, appearances can be deceptive. He combined intelligence with untrainability, and affection with ferocity. His deficiencies in conformation were dwarfed by his energy and tenacity. He ruled our family with a firm but benign paw.

Within a day of our adoption, he had mastered our swing-top garbage container. Placing the container in a cupboard slowed him not at all. A rubberband around the knobs on the paired doors fell in minutes to teeth and paws.

After enduring a floor covered with grapefruit rinds, apple cores, and coffee grounds, we bought a trash compactor. It was steel, and it had a pullout bin and a step-on latch. Moses watched us use the latch a few times, and soon the trash compactor yielded meekly to a step by his paw and a nudge with his nose. A bungee cord finally made our garbage secure.

Closed interior doors presented only a minor challenge. He quickly learned to twist the knob between his paws, pull or push, and get the door opened. This ability was especially a problem when guests arrived.

He could open the door leading to our patio, as well, and he let himself out whenever he wished. One afternoon, a telephone repair truck drove up to our back door. Moses woke from his nap, blasted out the door, and flew down the steps growling, barking, and salivating. The repairman jumped back into his truck, slammed the door, and rolled up the window. I secured Moses and went back outside. "The dog's locked up. You can come in now," I reassured him, through his cracked-open window.

"I think your trouble must be outside," he said.

Luckily, it was.

Moses was quite independent. Not only did he let himself out, but he soon learned to ring the doorbell. Initially, he scratched the door facing asking to come in. After accidentally hitting the doorbell and being admitted promptly, scratching was no longer necessary. If we were slow to answer, he just leaned on the bell button until we came.

Confinement was his greatest personal challenge. I built a five-foot-high chain-link fence to secure our three dogs, put Moses in the pen, latched the door… and he greeted me as I reached the house. He had simply put a paw through the gate and tripped the latch. I padlocked the gate, and he dug under. I stapled the fence to buried boards, and he climbed out. A wire roof finally secured him in the pen, but he never gave up—and broke most of his front teeth trying to chew through the steel wire.

Moses disliked baths. Our attempts to bathe him were futile, and as a last resort, we took him to a professional dog grooming service. When Carolyn arrived to take him home, the owner confessed, "He isn't here. I put him in a cage after his bath and in a few minutes, he strolled into my office. Not once in fifteen years have I failed to latch a cage, but there's always a first time. I put him back in the cage and made sure it was latched. He trotted into my office just as I reached my chair. The third time, I hid behind the door and watched. He lay on his back, put both paws through the bars, slid the bolt back and opened the door. He's now at the vet's next door in maximum security."

Moses died suddenly of an acute, massive intestinal hemorrhage.

He could not be replaced. We didn't try.

Birthdays, Anniversaries, and Such

The Brentwood Homepage will publish birthdays, anniversaries, and other significant days if they are significant enough. Recently, our fifty-third wedding anniversary has come and gone. And I even remembered it—and that is certainly significant. My forgetter is quite powerful. It overwhelms my rememberer quite regularly. But I exercise it much more, and so it keeps in good shape.

Of course, I have had little trouble remembering Christmas and Easter and Mother's Day. Modern merchandising sees to that. But birthdays and anniversaries don't enjoy such publicity. In my house, they come and go, often leaving the merest trace of a whimper. Carolyn bravely soldiers on without presents or cards or special nights out, and has stuck by me through fifty-three years of forgotten significant days. Is that why they call our spouses "significant others"?

I did remember our fiftieth wedding anniversary. We celebrated that one in year forty-nine. And in July, a month before our August date. Neither Carolyn nor I wanted huge formal reception/party/remarriage, or ceremony-type stuff. We decided on a family celebration, a celebration by the entire family—children, grandchildren, boyfriends, girlfriends. We decided to spend a week in the mountains.

And so our unofficial family social director, Tricia, began to plan. She spent hours on the Internet coordinating the festivities. The only time everyone could spare a week was in July. Since there were our three children and their spouses, eight grandchildren, and two serious girlfriends, we simply rented an entire small resort on a lake southeast of Chattanooga.

We rented a pontoon boat and two waverunners, and each family brought food for one supper. Breakfasts and lunches were supplied out of a common larder. Our grandchildren ranged in age from eight to twenty-one. We spent a week fishing, boating, waverunning, talking, laughing, and chasing the flock of Canada Geese away from our cabins.

We polished off huge amounts of food and soft drinks and bought about three-hundred dollars in gas for the boats. The weather was cool and dry, the fellowship was lively, and memories generated were indelible—especially of the geese.

Today and Many Yesterdays

Today is August tenth. Fifty-five years ago was much like today. It was a hot, cloudless day not marked by any major historic event. Even so, I should always remember it even though I have forgotten its significance once or twice. What's so great about the day fifty-five years ago? It was a life-changing day. It was the day Carolyn and I married.

I have told part of this story before, but I repeat it here. I had finished my second year in medical school and my roommate and I both had blind dates to some function, the type of which escapes me. I had a date with a quite forgettable girl, and my pal, Jimmy, had a date with Carolyn. She was the cutest, most attractive girl I had ever met. I thought, "I'd like to marry that girl."

Jimmy had a semi-steady girlfriend and was happy to allow me to call Carolyn for a date the next day. Though I was smitten, it took several months for Carolyn to become serious about me. We dated throughout my third year in medical school and married just before my senior year. I felt as though I had made the catch of the century.

Our marriage has survived the ups and downs of six long-distance moves, including a year in Sweden. We have survived the birth and rearing of three children, and have dealt with a few significant illnesses together.

Of course, there have been occasional disagreements. We have learned the necessity of give-and-take in our relationship and have learned the value of giving in. One day recently, Carolyn said, "I was really mad at you this week. I thought about what you did. Years ago I would have thought about divorce. Yesterday, I decided it wasn't too bad after all. We're not going to divorce at this late date so I just got over it."

No wonder I am still smitten.

I wrote this sonnet about five years ago, but it fits with anniversary memories today:

We gently kiss before we bed,
A thing we've done for fifty years.
It wipes away things best unsaid,
It dries up any burning tears.
We've lived for many, many years
Most of them as man and wife.
We've shed so very many tears,
We've shared a very happy life.
Happy night my dearest wife.
Who knows how many are to come?
If come joy or if come strife,
We will meet them both with calm.
We did a job that should be done,
To grow from two to be just one.

A Member of the Wedding

Almost everyone has been in weddings—some as the principal attraction, some in more minor roles.

I have participated in my share. I have been a groom only once, and that is all I ever intend to be. I have been groomsman, usher, best man, and father of the bride or groom, but never in the role I played last weekend. I was grandfather of the groom.

You may think the nuptial grandparent is a nothing job, and so did I—until last weekend. We thought, "All we have to do is to show up on time, be cordial and polite to everyone, keep any criticisms to ourselves, be escorted to our seats, sit still, hang around for pictures, hug the newly wedded couple, and keep still about our judgment that they are just too young for such a life-altering step."

However, as is common in these events, the unexpected intervened. The thinking went something like this: "Grandparents don't have anything to do. They'll be happy to…"

We delivered flowers, hors d'oeuvres, and cousins, among other chores. On Friday, the day before the wedding, we took one grandson-groomsman for a tux fitting, and transported three grandson members of the wedding to the rehearsal and the dinner afterward. We even took the engagement ring to the jewelers for cleaning on the morning of the wedding.

We, two ushers, and a groomsman, arrived early at the outdoor wedding venue and spent two hours fretting over the weather. (A late rainstorm would put an indelible imprint on the memories of the event.)

The setting was beautiful, the sky was clear, there was a gentle breeze, and the whole event came off as an almost seamless production.

Now that the birdseed blizzard has passed and their life together has begun, I hope that they will be able to attend a grandchild's wedding of their own one day.

Anna

Every child and every grandchild is special. I guess great-grandchildren are even extra-special. Maybe I will find out about that someday. Oldest and the youngest grandchildren are a bit extra-special as well, since they are the first and the last.

Anna is our youngest, a vibrant, feisty, saucy fourteen-year-old. I remember her younger days. First-grade teachers were faced with Anna's unique personality. It's not that Anna was a behavior problem—far from it. She was content to play for hours in an imaginary world with her dolls and stuffed toys. She was just not into rules. She could see no reason why she should color pictures within the lines if she felt coloring outside the lines would make a prettier picture. She lived in her own world. Adults were unwelcome. She saw no reason to change her attitude about her special world. Adults, keep out.

Some of her other ideas were a bit unusual, as well. She told me one summer that she would only wear flip-flops to first grade.

I asked, "Why?"

"I've forgotten how to tie my shoes."

"You can learn again."

"No, I can't. Learning to tie shoes was a kindergarten thing."

Anna and her mother spent the summer with us while Anna's mother recuperated from her fifth ankle surgery. One afternoon, Anna asked to make something in my woodworking shop. We decided to make an airplane. I crossed two scraps of soft white cedar to make a wing and a fuselage. I started four small nails and drove them through the wing part. I held the wing across the fuselage while Anna hammered the nails with a lightweight hammer. She tapped and tapped, very gently, making absolutely no progress. Finally, she looked up at me and, in a disgusted voice, complained, "Something is wrong with this hammer."

This last little vignette may have less to do with Anna's unique personality and more to do with the fact that all her cells all contain two X chromosomes. Anna's mother told six-year-old Anna that her other grandmother planned to take her shopping for school clothes the following day.

Anna stated firmly, "I'm glad I'm going with her. She might buy me something not in style."

A Family Crisis

Day One. Laura from daycare calls. "Anna has head lice. Come get her now! I tried to call her mother, her father, and her other grandparents. None of them answer!"

Carolyn replies, "It's four o'clock, and it takes us a half-hour to get there. Our daughter can pick her up at six o'lock."

"That's two hours! She has to leave now!"

Fifteen minutes on the phone results in an information-only call to her father, a warning call to our daughter, and a reassuring call to Laura.

Her mother is now on her way to pick up Anna and lice medicine. Whom in the family she will treat is still under discussion. Carolyn and I are standing by to provide daycare for little five-year-old, lice-afflicted Anna, should she need it.

Day two. Head treated, bedclothes and pajamas washed, hair thoroughly combed, no more nits seen, and it's off to school. Nits don't get past many kindergarten teachers, and the dreaded call comes, announcing our fates. "Nits."

What to do now? Shave her head? Fumigate the house? Burn it down? Homeschool her? Move, leaving no forwarding address? No one knows. A second treatment with a different medication and more combing are on the schedule for tonight. Perhaps she will have to forever wear a sign that says "UNCLEAN" as the biblical lepers did. Maybe she needs a miracle. This is worse than the ten plagues of Egypt! Where is Moses when you need him?

This scenario, with variations, has been repeated in hundreds of homes and plagued me for the twenty-five years of my pediatric practice. Nothing elicits more panic than head lice—unless it's pinworms. And neither one has ever caused anything worse than mild itching—on one end or the other.

Girls and Horses

What is it between girls and horses? I don't understand the attraction. Boats, I can understand. But then, there are some similarities between boats and horses. Both are expensive to buy, expensive to maintain the year round, and often require services of experts to repair damages to life, limb, hull, and sails. Of course, only horses leave evidence of their presence daily and spread it far and wide.

We can sit and admire horses and boats from near or far; we can caress them; we can groom them (and they seem to need grooming every day to look their best). I doubt grooming lends anything noticeable to their performance, but we seem to fully enjoy doing it as much as the object of our attention.

Our youngest daughter was born loving horses. She talked about horses with her first words. She began jumping horses in elementary school. I admit, her jumps were minimal at best, maybe a foot or so. But she jumped with the concentration and determination of the best show jumper. At four, she asked Santa for a saddle. When asked why, she replied, "To use on my white stallion when I get one next year."

She often stood at paddock fences admiring the horses. Often she would state, "That horse loves me." She took lessons for years, and of course, joined the Pony Club. She was limited to riding borrowed horses. It was not until she was in high school that we could afford a horse and his upkeep.

The horse came after more important toys—boats. I had coveted sailboats as long as I could remember. I never met a boat I didn't like. I guess my boat infatuation paralleled my daughter's horse attachment. I didn't buy my first boat until I was at least forty, when we could afford one without interrupting our retirement savings plan or borrowing money. It was an old nineteen-foot wooden sailboat built for racing. I learned how to sail in that boat. I even began to race a bit, but I never learned to sail fast. I seldom won. My only trophy is a third-place silver cup on display in one of our bathrooms.

Over the years I acquired a new (used) fiberglass boat of the same class and a new (new) small single hander.

Years passed, and the horse and my sailboats found new homes. I grew old; my daughter grew up. She has a daughter of her own who is a lover of horses. She rides, enters shows, and spends all day every Saturday in the horse barn grooming horses and cleaning stalls, a regular barn rat. She seems happiest with horse droppings on her boots.

What is it with girls and horses? She could be sailing.

Chapter Six, Memories of Growing Up

This section contains, without doubt, the most fiction of all the other sections. That said, many of these stories are true as I remember them. I will label each piece at the end of each story.

Of Frogs and Fire

When I was ten or so, I heard the story about how frogs react to change in temperature. As the story goes, if a person puts a frog in water and begins to heat the water very, very slowly, the frog will adapt to its environment so well that he will remain comfortable in the water until he is boiled to death.

I wondered about that. Could it be that the frog would just sit there as the water became warmer and warmer until he died? Maybe I would just test that story.

Step one: get a frog. That should not be a problem. There were plenty of frogs in the bayou, and the bayou was close by. All I needed was just one frog. Any size would do. I saw frogs everywhere in the bayou, but most were sunning themselves on logs several feet away from the bank—too far away for me to reach. The few frogs near the bank fled before I could get close enough to catch one.

I was stymied. What to do? I rode my bike back home and pondered my problem. I couldn't wade out to the frogs. They would be gone long before I reached them. I had no boat. What could I do? I needed a long-handled net—something that could reach a frog before he jumped into the water.

Our barn was a ready supplier of all manner of raw materials. I wired cheesecloth onto an old barrel hoop, and fastened the hoop to the end of a long bamboo pole. Now I had a catching tool that ought to work, though it looked like a butterfly net on steroids.

Back to the bayou. Have you ever looked at a frog up close? Ever notice those eyes? They stick out on the sides of their heads like horse droppings on a hard clay road. They are that way for a reason. It is hard to slip up on a frog—darn near impossible. They see everywhere, even behind their backs.

I could reach frogs easy enough—for what good it did. Those eyes picked up my weird frog catcher. No matter how quietly and slowly it approached a frog, off into the water he plopped. I worked all afternoon. Few frogs sunbathed that day, but many took a swim.

I just needed one frog—a dumb frog, a crippled frog—any kind of frog as long as he was alive. It took all afternoon, but finally I had my frog!

Step two: apply heat. I knew where I could do that, but when to do that was a problem. Mama had to be out of the kitchen, somewhere away from home. I knew she would not be quite as curious about frogs as I was—not nearly so curious, not even a little bit curious. But that's just how mothers are. They don't care much for frogs, but they do like a clean kitchen.

I was lucky. Mama was at the beauty shop that day. I pulled out a large pot, filled it about half full of water, and put it on the stove over a low flame. I plopped my frog in the pot, and splash! Out he jumped, doing what frogs do. He flopped around the kitchen, one flop ahead of this desperate scientist. I finally caught my subject and turned to start my experiment once again when Mama walked in. She looked at the stove, the pot, the poor frog in my fist and the water splotches on the floor.

"What is going on here?" Mama asked.

Things did look a bit unusual. Frogs had never lived in our house before. After a short lecture from Mama, I realized that frogs would never live here again.

I never did test the hypothesis about a frog in slowly warming water. Such are the frustrations of a research scientist.

This is pure fiction. I submitted it as part of my application for the Brentwood Homepage.

Armed and Dangerous

Everyone in town had a BB gun but me. Without arms, I risked becoming a social outcast, among the local ten-year-old set. Although all metal toys had disappeared from store shelves during World War II, a single BB gun appeared in the display window of Melton's General Store. I jumped on my bike, raced home, flew up the steps, and shouted, "Mama, Mama, Melton's has a BB gun! I need five dollars to buy it before someone else does."

To my surprise, Mama said, "Okay".

Owning a gun came with rules and responsibilities. "Do not shoot at anyone—ever. You could put an eye out." This was drilled into my head over and over. But I knew BB gun wars raged all over town, and no eyes had been put out so far.

One hot summer day my best friend, John, and I sat, slowly swinging on our porch.

"Nothing to do."

"Swimming?"

"Can't. Went day before yesterday. Nobody to take us."

"Fishing?"

"Too hot."

"Rubber guns?"

"Tired of that."

"BB gun fight?"

"Let's go."

We mounted our bikes and slipped out of the backyard, rode a mile down a forbidden major highway, and turned into the remains of an old sawmill—also forbidden territory. All that was left of the mill was a twenty-foot-high, half-acre sawdust pile. Winter rains had packed the sawdust rock-hard, and over many years, spontaneously-generated fires had created dozens of blackened chimneys, canyons, and caves. Several fires still smoldered and smoked.

I soon grew tired of hiding in caves and shooting (carefully aiming below the waist). To liven up the afternoon, I set an ambush. I picked out an especially good hiding place and lay in wait with my gun loaded, cocked, and ready. John's head appeared around a corner, and POW! I shot.

The loudest, shrillest, most out-of-this-world scream ever heard in three counties erupted from John's mouth. He clamped his hands over his face, jumped as high as he could, and spun round and round like a palsied ballerina shouting, "I'm shot! I'm shot! I'm shot!" I could see blood trickling between his fingers and running down his face.

I leapt out of my hiding place and ran toward him. "My God! My God! I've shot his eye out for sure! My BB gun is gone forever!" reverberated through my brain.

When John had calmed down a bit and I had screwed up my courage a bit, I pried his fingers off his face to assess the damage. Between his eyebrows, was a tiny, oozing, superficial puncture wound. Both eyes were miraculously intact!

Still, we had big problems. How could we explain that incriminating wound? At the forbidden sawdust pile? Down the forbidden highway? Finally, we concocted a far-fetched story of a freak bike wreck.

Another miracle happened that day. Our parents believed us.

This is one of my memories from childhood. It is as close to true as I can remember.

Being a Bird

I can fly, not like a bird, but I can fly. I can fly, if I have an airplane around me. I can fly, if the engine runs, if the propeller turns, and if the wings don't fall off. I need an instructor beside me as well.

I don't have a license. I am too old to pass the physical, and it is too expensive to complete pilot training. Instead, I fly once or twice a year with someone who knows what he is doing. I can take off. Landings are still scary. If conditions are not ideal, pilot friends do the landings.

My first flying experience occurred when I was about thirteen. I hung around a crop duster's airfield doing odd jobs, hoping for a ride. Toward the end of the crop dusting season, the owner of the service invited me up for a flight in his two-seater airplane. This was his personal plane, not a duster. Dusters held only the pilot and a ton or so of insecticide.

We strapped in and the pilot flipped a switch, pushed the starter button, and pushed the throttle forward. The engine caught, stuttered, spit smoke from the exhaust pipes. He adjusted the fuel mixer, and the engine settled down to a smooth cadence. The ground crew removed the wheel chocks, the pilot pushed the throttle a bit forward, and we bounced along the ground toward the grass-covered landing strip.

When we reached the leeward end of the strip, he turned our plane into the wind and revved the engine to its maximum speed, and we trundled down the bumpy track. We left the earth about halfway down. We were not loaded down with cargo the way the dusters were. It was just the two of us. We climbed toward the south for several minutes, made a climbing turn toward the west, and leveled out at about two thousand feet. The plane was noisy, much more so than I had imagined, but I didn't care. I was flying. Maybe not like a bird, but here I was where the birds were—high in the sky.

It was more than I had ever hoped for. And then, my pilot friend said, "Take the yoke. Do you know what the yoke and foot pedals do?"

Of course I did. I had loved flying since I could remember, even though it was a vicarious love. I had built dozens of model planes, flown the better ones, had even designed planes of my own (though they invariably were disasters). I knew about control surfaces. Yoke and rudder pedals were child stuff. I had read every book on flying I could lay my hands on.

"Then take the yoke!" he shouted over the engine noise.

And take the yoke and rudder pedals I did. I climbed gently, dove gently, and turned right and left ever so gently, knowing a steep turn would cause a loss of altitude. I turned and rose and dipped and turned until I could do no more. He talked me through the landing sequence: the upwind leg, the crosswind leg, the downwind leg, the final leg, and the descent to the runway.

He said, "You handle the plane very well. Do you want to land it?"

Heavens no! I might crash it. "No. You land it." And he did.

The afternoon was pay enough for the summer I spent picking up trash and washing planes.

I had flown.

Part fiction, part true.

Part-Time Jobs

I never received an allowance until I reached college. I earned my spending money.

I delivered milk. Though we lived in town, we had a barn and pasture with dairy cows. We used the milk for ourselves and to sell for extra money. My father gave me a six-house milk route when I started first grade. My dog, Skippy, and I delivered milk twice a week. Skippy exuded an officious sense of importance as he led me to each house. I earned twenty-five cents a week from my route. Not big money to you, but plenty for a six-year-old in the 1930s.

My father and great-uncle owned a busy cotton business. They bought raw cotton from farmers in Mississippi, Louisiana, and sometimes Texas and supplied cotton to mills throughout the South.

They employed several office workers to process their purchases and sales. Beginning in the eighth grade, I was the janitor. I worked every morning before school and was the errand boy on Saturdays and days off. I never learned to classify the large number of cotton types each farmer grew, but I did learn a bit about how to deal with people.

I loved to watch my great-uncle deal with farmers offering to sell their crops. I usually found some dusting or sweeping to do in the sample room while Uncle Robert dealt with a farmer. Some would bring in all the cotton samples and say, "Here's my crop. I'll pick up my check tomorrow." Others would haggle for hours, sometimes even taking their samples to another broker and returning later.

I asked my great-uncle, "Why is it that you give the same price to both farmers?"

He replied, "Some like to haggle; some don't. They both get a fair price."

But cotton merchants had no work in summers, when crops were immature and all sales had been delivered. I realized I needed a summer job.

I applied for a job as helper in a carpenter crew. I was hired on a trial basis, to be on probation for two weeks. The first day, I watched the other helper, a crippled black man at least seventy years old. I reasoned that if I kept up with him, I would qualify to work the entire summer. That old man worked slowly and steadily all eight hours, and I kept up—but just barely.

I did the usual helper things, carrying lumber and bricks and bundles of roofing shingles. I helped dig foundation footings, pushed a wheelbarrow, and picked up trash around the construction site.

I had one job that was mine alone—making coffee for our midmorning break. One morning on a new project in the countryside, I realized there was no source of water. I approached the boss and said, "We don't have water for coffee. Do you want to drive to town for some water?"

"No. Just use some from the barrel we washed our shovels in this morning. The dirt should be settled by now."

And that's what I did. The coffee tasted a bit strange and little gritty but we drank it.

This is a small sample of my temporary jobs. I had a total of seven jobs while growing up in Mississippi. I earned my spending money and more besides; more importantly, I learned something about the world and people in it, and kept a great suntan all summer long.

It's a shame kids are deprived of summer jobs these days.

All true as I remember it.

Uncle Robert's Commissary

When I was a young boy a long, long time ago, Uncle Robert had a commissary.

He was my great-uncle, the brother of my paternal grandmother. My daddy and Uncle Robert were partners in business. They owned and ran a cotton trading company. It was quite successful and occupied most of my father's time and energy—but not Uncle Robert's.

Uncle Robert owned quite a number of other businesses. He had three large cotton farms, had the cotton company, was a major stockholder in several small banks, engaged in several real estate ventures with his brother, and partnered with a large cotton company in Memphis. One unusual business he had was a commissary for use by the employees of his farms.

His commissary was very similar to a country general store. He sold canned goods, meats, some produce, and dry goods. He also stocked an assortment of tobacco products, including chewing tobacco and snuff and small bags of tobacco for roll-your-own cigarettes.

He also had a stock of caskets. I don't remember any other retailer of caskets in the Mississippi Delta country outside of funeral homes, but Uncle Robert had a large inventory of an inexpensive line of caskets.

Uncle Robert also had a large stock of stories, some of which were probably true. He could be counted on to tell stories appropriate for any occasion at every family gathering. I will never forget one story he told about the caskets.

During the Great Depression of the 1930s few people had money—hardly enough for basic necessities. Because so little cash was available, many transactions were on the barter system. A very poor man lost his wife and had no money for a casket. He struck a bargain with Uncle Robert for his cheapest casket in exchange for a calf just born on his farm. The calf was to be delivered when it had been weaned.

Uncle Robert said, "The farmer finally delivered my calf. She was the scrawniest bovine I had ever seen. I thought about grabbing her by the tail and slinging her over the fence and back in the farmer's face, but I was afraid her tail might come off. And a deal's a deal, so I took the calf.

"Do you know what? That calf grew unto a great large cow, and she gave more milk than any cow I ever had. A deal's a deal. That deal turned out to be a good one."

All true.

Don't Tread on Me

"When frost is on the pumpkin and corn is in the shock..." (James Whitcomb Riley)

My family owned a small cotton farm three miles from our home in the Mississippi Delta. My brother-in-law managed our farm and two other rented farms.

One of our income sidelines was growing high-quality paper-shell pecans. We had a twenty-acre grove in an area poorly adapted for cotton or other row crops. The trees were fertilized once or twice a year, and the grove was disked periodically for weed control. The only other activity was the harvest in late fall.

Though they required minimal care, and in good years, provided a welcomed added income, there was one chronic problem: It seems that almost everyone considers nut trees to be in the public domain and available to all without charge. Simply pick them up, bag them up, and go on your merry way.

My brother-in-law had a different idea. He felt the pecans were his. They grew on his land; he fertilized them; he kept the weeds down; he deserved the profit from them.

One late fall day, my brother-in-law saw a strange pickup truck parked on the far side of his pecan grove. There was a man with a tow sack in the grove busily picking up pecans. There was a full sack in the truck bed.

My brother-in-law slipped to the pickup and removed the valve stems from all four tires.

In an hour or so, the dusty, sweaty poacher approached my brother-in-law at our barn and said, "Could I borrow your air tank and four valve stems? Somebody stole all four of my valve stems from my truck."

My brother-in-law said, "I won't lend you any stems, but I'll sell you these four for those pecans of mine in your truck."

His motto could very well have been, "Don't tread on me—or my pecan grove."

All true.

Cucumbers

Our local daily paper ran a story several months ago on the climate bill passed by the House of Representatives. The program would allow utilities and other polluters to comply with greenhouse gas emission rules by buying credits from farmers who plant trees on their property. The new law reminded me of another law designed to limit production of crops on the federal price-support lists.

Farmers are a resourceful lot. They adapt to changing weather, changing market prices, changing farming techniques, and changing federal laws and regulations. I wonder how they would adjust to the cap-and-trade law if it were passed.

In the 1950s, federal price supports changed. Instead of limiting the acreage allowed to be planted in a certain crop (cotton, where I grew up), Congress enacted a law requiring farmers to set aside acreage to lie fallow, growing nothing for a season. The land had to be kept weed-free, but no crops could be produced. Of course, there were exceptions. One exception was cucumbers. Farmers were allowed to grow cucumbers on "set aside" land without penalty.

My cousin decided to do just that. He planted a twenty-acre field in cucumbers.

He signed a contract with a pickle factory in a nearby town, and began his harvest in June. Twenty pickers harvested a truckload of cucumbers every day, six days a week. The cucumbers in that field were more than enough to supply fresh slices to every salad—and pickles for every sandwich—in the entire state of Mississippi. He spent most of every day trucking cucumbers, unloading them, and returning his empty truck to the field. This went on all summer long. Not until late September was the harvest finished.

When I returned from college at Christmastime, I asked him how he did with his cucumbers.

He replied, "I did very well. I almost broke even."

I wonder if cucumbers might beat trees as a friend of the environment and the farmer, too. At least the farmer could hope to break even.

A true story.

The Last Great Indian Uprising

When Uncle Robert was a young boy, he lived on a farm a short distance from the small town of Earlsboro in the Oklahoma Territory. His family included his two older sisters, Etta (my grandmother) and Maud (the oldest). They attended a one-room school some two to four miles from their home. Uncle Robert, by his own admission, was a short, chubby five or six year old at the time of this story.

One hot autumn day, a rider galloped up to the school on a heaving, lathered horse. He jumped off before the horse had completely stopped, and he landed in a cloud of dust shouting, "Indian raid! Indian raid! Get home as quick as you can!"

Children grabbed books, lunch pails, and hats, and started for home. Robert, Etta, and Maud streaked for home, running through fields, woods, and ditches because they were afraid Indians were watching the roads. Soon Uncle Robert's, short legs and chubby belly betrayed him. He ran slower and slower, fell farther and farther behind, and finally, sat down unable to take another step. Maud stopped, came back, picked up Robert, put him on her back, and carried him the rest of the way home.

At home, they found their parents throwing guns, ammunition, flour, hams, coffee, sugar, quilts, lanterns, skillets, plates, and cups into their two-horse wagon. Their father shouted, "Get in the wagon quick!" He slapped the horses and off they flew, with two dogs following close behind.

The courthouse in Earlsboro was engulfed in barking dogs, horses, crying babies, cursing men, somber women, and dust. Soon, the doors and windows were fortified with bags of flour and bales of hay. Coffee boiled, babies cried and nursed, men walked about looking grim, women whispered to each other and worried, and children played, fought, and generally disrupted the solemnity of the occasion.

As night fell, the men watched at the fortified windows, children slept on quilt pallets, and women talked in whispers. All the dogs were kept outside so that their barking might alert the garrison of any night attack.

It was a long night. At dawn, a solitary rider slowly rode up to the courthouse, dismounted somewhat stiffly, ambled up the courthouse steps, and announced, "The uprising's off. It was only one Indian with too much to drink, shooting at clouds."

And so, the "Last Great Oklahoma Indian Uprising" ended not in a massacre, but in a whimper.

My Great Uncle Robert was the family storyteller. He claims this story is true—at least the bare-bones plot. Most, if not all, embellishments are fiction.

Distemper

About three months ago, I mentioned my Kindle reader Christmas present. I have enjoyed playing with my new toy and have ordered several books. Recently, Amazon displayed a list of one hundred books priced at less than three dollars each. I scrolled through the list and ordered a book by James Herriot, the English veterinarian and author.

I think it was his last book. As usual, it deals with episodes in his practice. One of his stories dealt with an epidemic of distemper among the dogs in his area. He describes the intestinal symptoms, the severe cough and nasal discharge, the weight loss and severe loss of appetite followed by seizures, and often, death. Dogs seldom recover from this devastating viral illness.

Fortunately, potent vaccines are available now, and I doubt the vets see distemper among domesticated dogs today. I would guess it still ravages wild animal populations.

I experienced distemper only once. I was given a rat terrier puppy when I was six years old. This was before the vaccine was available, and Skippy developed distemper when he was only a few months old. He developed the typical symptoms of runny nose and eyes, cough, loss of appetite, and weight loss.

Our veterinarian suggested a series of symptomatic measures and warned us of the serious and likely fatal course we could expect. Despite our best efforts, Skippy became worse. He could hardly rise from his bed and had stopped eating. The vet came again and pronounced Skippy's fate once again. He suggested, as a last-ditch effort, to offer him some eggnog to tempt him to eat something, no matter how little.

My parents were strict teetotalers, so of course, there was no whiskey in the house. Daddy sneaked into the local bootlegger's establishment and bought a pint of the best bourbon available. (If Skippy was going to Hell for drinking, he might as well go first class.) Daddy slipped the bottle into his pocket and drove straight home, hoping to avoid meeting any friends along the way.

Mama stirred up a batch of eggnog and carefully poured a tablespoon of whiskey into the mixture. Daddy added a generous dollop more—enough to do some good, he said. Skippy sniffed the drink, took a few tentative licks, then emptied the bowl, stood up, let out an ear-rattling howl, and sat beside the bowl begging for more.

Skippy was cured! He rapidly regained his appetite and weight, and his respiratory symptoms abated. He was only left with a susceptibility to bronchitis every winter and a daily futile search for eggnog.

True as I remember it. Facts confirmed by my older sister.

The Calf

When I was eleven or twelve years old, I developed an itch to raise a beef cow. Several of my schoolmates had bragged about how much money they made raising calves for meat. Easy money! Just turn the calf out in the pasture, wait about nine or ten months, sell the cow to the packinghouse, then go home and count your money.

I pestered Daddy endlessly for a calf. Finally, he relented and gave me a young bull calf. We had a half-acre paddock beside our house that contained a milk cow and chickens. We trucked the calf to our home "pasture," and the calf was mine to care for and to profit from. Unfortunately, the pasture was too small to support both the calf and our milk cow, so we bought hay. The calf got sick, and the vet came. It was unusually cold that winter, and I often had to break ice in the water trough and give him extra feed. In spite of my exemplary care, he loved to surprise me with a friendly butt into my backsides. I did not regard it as a sign of affection.

Every morning I got up early, ate breakfast, fed and watered the calf, cleaned Daddy's office, and then went to school. This calf was not a pet—not even close. I rapidly became sick of the whole project. As soon as the calf was big enough, off to the packinghouse he went. The next day I picked up my check, and the numbers on the check almost made my winter's travails bearable.

Daddy then pulled out small book. He had, unknown to me, kept a list of all of my expenses. He started subtracting, and subtracting, and kept on subtracting.

Finally, after my profit had shrunk to exactly one-dollar-and-fifty cents, I looked up at him and said, "Daddy, I am no longer in the cow business!"

A true story. I left the cattle business for medicine, without regret.

The Tuesday Garden Club

The first Tuesday of the month was holy. The garden club met that day. Nothing could interfere with the garden club. Weddings were always on Saturdays, so they were never a problem. Occasionally a funeral did interfere, often because there was a new pastor in town—usually a Methodist. Methodist pastors came and went every few years at the whim of the bishop, and it took a while for each new one to discover how things were done here. After two Tuesday funerals, someone in the club always saw to it that the new pastor was gone within the year—and with good riddance.

Nobody crossed the garden club, no matter how good were his sermons or his intentions. Not even the bishop could stand up to the garden club.

The commandment, "Thou shalt keep the first Tuesday of the month holy. It shalt not be defiled by weddings, funerals, other club meetings, school plays, or ballgames," must be in the Bible somewhere, though it is hard to find. I think it may be in the seventeenth chapter of Mark, but I am not sure.

The club tolerated acts of God on first Tuesdays, even though they had not been sanctioned by a committee. No officer had yet discovered how to persuade God never to schedule rainstorms, tornadoes, floods, or snowfalls on the first Tuesdays of the month. Ever tolerant, the club never chastised God for such lapses, though there was a sizable minority who would have liked to have done so.

The club was limited to twelve—not by rule, but by custom. Most active members were ladies in their forties or fifties. There were a few older ones who still held unofficial honorary membership. They did not have to host the club in their homes, make refreshments, or arrange a program. Mostly, what they did was to have given birth to a future club member and to have survived into their seventies.

Young matrons waited for older members to die or become inactive so that they could assume their rightful place. New member orientations were unnecessary. Every woman of that standing had the rules of etiquette embedded in her DNA, inherited through her mother's X chromosome. They were born knowing Southern Small Town Social Graces.

Although it was called a "garden club," not one member had ever made compost, planted a bulb or a seed, pulled a weed, or dug up sod for a new flowerbed. Their black yardmen did all that. The most work the ladies did was to pat the perspiration from their foreheads while they picked an occasional bouquet. They preferred to make fancy arrangements of the flowers their yardmen had picked.

Hot, dirty, grubby toil did not fit their lifestyle. It might mess up their hair.

This story is a product of some of my memories, liberally laced with fiction.

Bugs

It's summertime, time for heat, time for vacation, time for swimming, time for sunburn, and time for bugs.

This year is the time for cicadas. Just like Old Faithful in Yellowstone National Park, one can count on their appearance. But unlike the hourly eruption of water, cicadas in Middle Tennessee explode only every thirteen years. They compress a life of hatching, molting, mating, egg laying, and dying into only a day or so. But they are a nuisance during that time. We are left with cleaning up dead bugs and empty shells, but after a few weeks of nuisance they are gone.

I grew in the Mississippi Delta, a land of flat fields, of bayous and swampy places—a land of farms, a land of bugs. Mosquitoes approached giant size most years. They were not quite as big as hummingbirds, but they could challenge cicadas for size. They were said to carry off small calves and large children, but I have never seen that. My great-uncle had said more than once he saw four average-size mosquitoes carry off a small child. I have my doubts about that. He is prone to exaggerate. There may have been more than four.

But of all the buggy nuisances in the Delta, chiggers were the worst—hands down. It's not that they are so big; they're not. It's just that they are so many of them. And they are so vicious. I've never seen a person lose enough blood to the little suckers to harm him, but it's not from their lack of trying.

I can never forget the chigger infestations when I was a child. They itch like crazy, and I defy any six-year-old to go five minutes without scratching. They congregate in areas of tight-fitting clothing such as underwear briefs, making scratching something of an antisocial exercise. But scratch we did.

Daddy had a surefire cure for chiggers. He doused the affected parts with a liberal splash of rubbing alcohol. It burned like stepping on a red-hot horseshoe, but it totally eliminated the itchiness. One dose cured.

If it didn't, nobody let on. We just didn't scratch.

The truth of the mosquito story is high suspect. However, I stand as proof of the efficiency of Daddy's chigger therapy.

Cafés

Our town had no restaurants You had to go over thirty miles for one of those. We did have cafés. We had hamburger joints, meat-and-threes, tearooms, and sandwich and soda fountains in the drug store. Of course, not all the cafés were here at the same time. They seemed to open, enjoy success when new, do a few months of so-so business, and then have a decline, either slow or fast, depending on the quality of the food.

There was little variation in the quality of the service, the décor, or the cleanliness of the place. The first was casual but efficient, the second was haphazard, the third was marginal at best.

Only the bravest of the brave opened a tearoom. They had to have been financially backed better than anyone to have a chance to remain open longer than a month or so. Only ladies of the garden club, Bible study groups, book club, or DAR would ever be caught in a tearoom. No matter how tasty the cucumber sandwiches and salads were, no self-respecting male would ever enter such an establishment. It was doomed from its birth.

A pizzeria opened in our town. It was part of a chain. How it got in our town remains a mystery. It lasted less than a year. Once, when I ordered a large pizza with half mushrooms, half sausage, I was met by the question, "Which half do you want the mushrooms on?" With servers like that, one wonders what is going on in the kitchen.

The pizzeria didn't last long. I think it was that small town rural Mississippi was not ready for prepackaged "Italian" food. Our Italian cafés served authentic Italian fare. They would not even have let a pizza occupy space in their dumpster out back.

Most of our cafés were meat-and-threes. Over the years, they came and went. Most had good greasy meat dishes, canned vegetables enhanced by added grease, wonderful greasy cornbread, and pies and cakes made on the premises. Cholesterol and calories hadn't been invented yet.

One day my great-uncle took an out-of-town client to lunch at our local meat-and-three. (Aunt Nora was out of town, or she would have put a gourmet Southern meal on the table.) Uncle Robert and his client looked over the menu—a pretty standard offering.

The client ordered, among other things, a salad. He asked his waitress, "What salad dressings do you have?"

"We have every salad dressing there is."

"I'll have Roquefort."

"We don't have that."

And that's the way cafés were where I grew up.

An amalgam of all the cafés I patronized in my youth.

Night at Grandma and Grandpa's House

August was a special time—the month we spent two weeks at Grandma and Grandpa's house in Oklahoma. My first memory of those visits was when I was five years old.

Grandma and Grandpa's house had three bedrooms, one bathroom, a living room, and dining room and kitchen—the usual arrangement of houses built in the 1920s. Unlike most houses, it had a bonus room, a Florida room. It was located on the southwest corner of the house and had windows across the entire two outside walls. The room contained a couch that unfolded into a bed. The bed was hard and lumpy, suitable only for five-year-olds. That was where I slept. I had no problem with sleeping in the Florida room—until I went to bed.

Oklahoma plains are known for their winds. They blow every day, and strongly. Fifteen-to twenty-mile-per-hour winds were common. People seldom mentioned the wind until it blew thirty or more.

At bedtime, later than usual because I was on vacation, Mama opened the couch, made up my bed, and tucked the sheet under my chin. All the windows in the room were open. The dry, nighttime breeze cooled the room nicely. (There were no air-conditioned houses in the 1930s.)

Light from a full moon streamed into the room, making almost enough light to read by. Mama gave me a goodnight kiss and turned off the light as she left the room.

Grownups complain about trouble sleeping in a strange bed. Children don't. We can sleep anywhere—so they say. Maybe it was the strange bed, maybe it was because of the excitement of the day, maybe it was something else, but I did not drop off to sleep immediately. I tossed and turned, pulled my sheet this way and that, and flopped over one way and back again. Sleep would not come.

I heard a weird moaning sound. It waxed louder, abated, returned louder than ever, ebbed, became louder, then grew softer, but never stopped. I opened my eyes and looked out. There, just outside the windows on the west wall, strange, dark, saucer-sized shapes danced in the air. They fluttered and spun and soared and returned in a terrifying way. Sometimes they looked like spear points. Then they changed to thin streaks. The swishing, moaning sound was coming from those dancing shapes. There had to be some kind of monster, an evil thing, with its eye on ME! It had to be. Evil monsters were after me! I was doomed! I pulled the sheet over my head, curled into a tight ball, closed my eyes, and lay as still as a corpse. I went to sleep that way, knowing this night was likely my last night on earth.

I woke early, alive, every part of my body intact. I had survived the night. I had beaten the evil forces outside. I shed my pajamas, pulled on my shorts and shirt, ran outside, and cautiously crept around the corner of the house where my sleeping room lay. There stood a catalpa tree just outside the windows of my room. Its large leaves rustled in the wind, fluttering and spinning and soaring and returning and rising and falling—just the way big leaves do in the wind. Just the way they had the previous night.

I had found my evil monster. I never told Mama or Daddy or Grandma or Grandpa, and especially not my older sister and my two snotty older cousins. I slept very well every night the rest of the two weeks.

Such are the exaggerated imaginings of young children. What I saw was very real to me—just misinterpreted.

Communications

Our little Southern town was part of the vast information network of the entire country. And we could surely spread the news, almost as quick then as now, even without email, spam, blogs, or Facebook.

We had a post office. It was located only a block from the railroad depot. Of course, most everything else was not too far from there, either. Cotton fields began not five blocks away.

Mail came by train, three times a day. People met the mail train if they expected an important letter or package. There was no home delivery, but mail was in the post office, sorted and ready for pick after every train run—this for a three-cent stamp for first class letters and a one-cent stamp for postcards, each of which the postmaster felt duty-bound to read.

❧

Our town was progressive. We had telephone service—maybe "service" is a little bit pretentious. There were only a hundred or so of us with a phone. Our sets were mounted on the wall in a hallway or some other central place. Nobody had more than one, not even the doctor. The phone was a wooden box about the size of a breadbox with a speaker poking out the front, an earpiece hanging on the left, and a crank on the right. To make a call, we lifted the earpiece, cranked the crank, and told the switchboard operator, "Bertie, I need to talk to Mr. Jones." Bertie did it if she could.

Sometimes, she would say, "Mr. Jones is over at the Whitworth's. I'll ring him there."

We had private lines, not party lines. But still, Bertie knew everything and enjoyed keeping the town informed of the goings-on of its leading citizens.

Nobody wanted to make Bertie mad.

Mr. Fowler owned our phone system, not the Bell Telephone. He owned the household sets, the telephone exchange, the wires, the poles, and their insulators—everything. Bertie closed down the exchange at nine o'clock every night.

We had no service on Sundays. Who could expect someone to work at night or on a Sunday just for calls? If you needed a doctor or the night watchman or the pharmacist after nine or on a Sunday, you went to get him. That's just the way it was. Nobody thought anything about it.

Rainy days were a trial. There were glass insulators made just for phone lines, but we kids loved to use them as targets for our new .22 rifles. Mr. Fowler replaced the broken ones with Coke bottles. They were glass, had an indentation in their middles to tie a line on, and were hollow (so they could be stuck on a sharp stick attached to a pole, a tree, or even to a fence post), and they were free. They worked very well if installed just right, but Mr. Fowler wasn't too particular about where he attached the bottles—or, for that matter, how he attached them.

Rainstorms played havoc with the phone service. Lots and lots of places shorted out with just a heavy dew. Mr. Fowler never got too excited about the phone service in rainy weather. He could get out and slog through the mud in the woods and the fields and wade the surging water in ditches to fix the lines, or he could go coon hunting for a couple of days and dry weather would fix the lines for him. Dry weather won out every time.

Yes, we had all the modern conveniences—mail service, telephones, our weekly newspaper—but none of these could match the real local news. Some might call it gossip. Within an hour of its occurrence, news of a birth, a death, a family squabble, a bankruptcy, a financial killing, a people killing, or even a new car became common knowledge all over town.

Even with editorial additions, you could count on the accuracy of oral news above that of the weekly newspaper. And it was certainly faster.

We adolescents hated the oral news. It left very little room for misbehavior. Mama seemed to know everything I did before I got home.

This story is mostly true. I have changed the names to protect the innocent.

Chapter Seven, Home and Food

I have placed these topics together. Who can separate home and food—at least in a Southern kitchen of the mid-twentieth century?

Dwelling Places

A holly tree grows beside our deck. Mockingbirds have nested in the tree for the entire thirty-seven years we have lived here. It can't be the same bird, of course. She doesn't wear glasses or fly with a cane. I think it must be one of her great-great-granddaughters or something.

People love mockingbirds and protect them despite their fierce territorial instinct. They will attack other birds, and also dogs and cats and humans who are perceived a threat to their nests. Don't mess with a mockingbird protecting her tree. Our beagle can testify to that.

Once a year, a flock of about one-hundred robins descend on the holly tree, intent on eating the ripe red berries. The resident mockingbird charges from side to side, squawking and flapping her wings trying to scare the robins away. As soon as she squawks at one side, robins fly to the other side, evading the mockingbird at every turn. The poor mockingbird needs resuscitation and counseling once the robins have stripped the tree and sought other luncheon sites.

Skunks are a different matter. Females make dens. A favorite place is under the slab that supports our air conditioner. Often, they will dig a den so deep that it opens underneath the house. We had that problem one summer.

Mama skunk dug herself a first-class maternity ward. Soon, there were seven juniors occupying the den. Needless to say, we easily nosed them out. I trapped all eight. Employees of the Williamson County Animal

Control and I became well-acquainted that summer. I trapped; they carried the skunks off in my Haveaheart trap. They were sprayed only once. They must really know their business to deal with skunks every day and still be allowed to come home at night.

I have a live-and-let-live relationship with mockingbirds. Don't bother me, and I won't bother you.

Skunks are a different matter. Our skunk maternity ward is closed. If there is a repeat, I may try to sell our house to a buyer with a bad sinus condition.

Shade Tree Plumber

I can do almost anything around the house. I can hang doors, build shelves and clothes hampers, replace faucet washers and light bulbs, even hang pictures and wallpaper with the help of a good marriage counselor.

I can replace light switches, doorbell chimes, and commode flap valves. DVD players and VCRs no longer intimidate me—very much.

I can paint, though very reluctantly and sloppily—so sloppily that Carolyn doesn't ask me to paint anymore.

Once, I was a handyman plumber. I could cut iron pipe, cut threads, and join pipe together with iron connectors. My propane torch, flux, and solder overwhelmed any defenses copper tubing might mount to defeat a soldered joint.

Plumbing presented little challenge to this backyard pipe fitter—or so I thought. Then it happened. The shutoff valve in our master bathroom commode tank failed. A fine spray of water began to issue from the valve area. No amount of shaking or pounding lessened the stream. It flowed on and on, oblivious to my ministrations.

It was obvious that a new valve mechanism was needed. I looked the problem over with an "expert" eye. The plastic thing with the valve and float just screws into the bottom of the tank. I could replace the whole mechanism in just a few minutes. No need to call our plumber. No need to pay a big fee. Since it happened on a Saturday, I could take care of this myself.

I left the hardware store with a shiny new plastic valve mechanism that the salesman assured me would fit every commode tank in existence. (I go to the hardware store so often that I have earned "frequent shopper miles" with an automatic ten-percent discount on everything I buy.)

Back home once again, I removed the tank lid. Too bad, the valve had not cured itself.

I attacked the problem in my usual organized manner.

Step one: Turn off the water.

Step two: Remove the old valve mechanism. Step three: Install the new mechanism.

Step four: Turn on the water. Step five: Admire my plumbing skills.

I got as far as step one. The shutoff valve beneath the commode presented a problem. As soon as I turned the knob, a stream issued from around the shutoff stem. Water flowed in a steady drip, drip, drip. What to do? Open the valve? Maybe the leak would stop. No luck. It flowed, drip, drip, drip. What to do? Put a pan under it? We can't have water all over the bathroom floor. The valve is only two inches above the floor. Only a pie pan would fit. How long before the pan would be full? No longer than an hour.

It was a Saturday morning. Monday was two days away. I would have to empty the pan every hour for two days. That was indeed a problem. How to solve it? Turn off the water to the entire house at the street? Not a solution. Call our plumber? A practical, but painful, solution. Nothing else to do. Call Mr. Feinstein.

He came that afternoon, replaced the valve at the floor, replaced the shutoff valve in the tank, and presented me with a bill with a one-hundred-dollar surcharge for weekend work.

He told Carolyn, "Let me do the plumbing, and let the doctor do the doctoring."

I took his advice and resigned from the plumbing fraternity. Plumbing is no longer in my home-repairman repertoire.

The Handyman

As long as I can remember, I have been the one called upon to fix things. My father was a successful businessman and an outstanding athlete, but he was no handyman. He passed along every household repair to me, claiming—with some validity—that his hands were too valuable to risk in household repairs. He was an expert classer of raw cotton, able to measure fiber length to a thirty-secondth inch by feel alone. That was part of how he made his living.

I am self-taught in various home repair skills. I can rewire lamps, replace electrical outlets and plugs, repair valves and washers in commodes, and other simple repairs. Of course, I carried these skills over into married life and have kept our house more or less functional through fifty-five years.

Some chores have required less skill and more brute persistence. I remember the call at our hotel room at a regatta when our children were small. We called home after the first day on the water and were reassured that all was well at home—until our youngest began to speak.

She said, "Our toothbrushes melted when we boiled them, but the hairbrush is okay."

That brought an immediate request to talk to the woman who was supervising our household while Carolyn and I were sailing. We learned the bathroom over our garage had been invaded by thousands of mites that had migrated up the wall from an abandoned starling nest.

As soon as we returned home, I realized the nest must go. I cut through the drywall ceiling and pulled out a wastebasket-full of bird nest materials. Fortunately, the birds had all flown away. A large patch fashioned from a scrap of drywall ended the nesting problem.

We bought a used refrigerator early in our marriage. It served us faithfully for years, though its appearance was less than ideal. After several years, it began to cool food poorly. I checked the refrigerator and found a solution. The button that turns the interior light off had become so worn that it made poor contact with the door and let cold air escape. I taped a soda-bottle cap to the door, and contact was restored. Carolyn was less than happy. She already had plans to pick out a new refrigerator.

Last week, the sensor for the front door began to fail. I kicked the door, opened it and slammed it shut, and the sensor failed to respond. As a last resort, I gave it a sharp rap with my screwdriver handle and the sensor once again functioned well— intermittently.

Carolyn asked, "Are you going to hang the screwdriver by the door or use a bottle cap?"

I called the security company.

Pets

Almost every family has had pets at one time or another. Our family is no exception. Of course, we had dogs and cats. We had one of the world's smartest dogs and one of the world's dumbest cats. You have read about our genius dog, Moses, who, among other self-taught accomplishments, could let himself out and ring the doorbell to be let in.

We had other pets as well. I do not consider as pets the kindergarten parakeet that died while we were caring for him over the Christmas holiday, or the lizard Bill caught at YMCA day camp that starved, because we could not catch enough live flies, the only thing he would eat.

When the children were in elementary school, we finally relented to persistent pleas and bought a gerbil and a hamster. I bought a cage for the hamster, but I used a small, cracked aquarium for the gerbil. I reasoned that nothing could climb those vertical, smooth glass walls.

He escaped the first night.

My daughter, Cathy, checked on her new pet at three a.m., found him missing and woke her mother, who kicked me out of bed, threatening me with severe bodily harm if that gerbil remained a fugitive. Even though Carolyn weighed only one hundred pounds, I was afraid to test her resolve when I saw that steely look in her eyes. I found the gerbil in the far corner of a closet, put him back in his aquarium, covered it with a heavy book, and slipped back into bed. I made a hardware cloth cover for the aquarium that afternoon.

A few weeks later, Carolyn took a weekend sabbatical with her buddies at Red Boiling Springs, a nearby old resort, where they played bridge for twelve hours a day. Cathy took her gerbil out of his cage to play with him. He tried to escape, and Cathy grabbed him by his tail. The furry tuft came off in her hand and I had to chase him down again, bloody tail and all. A quick exam revealed about a half inch of exposed tailbone. If the bone were left uncovered, it would become infected, ultimately leading to the gerbil's demise. Amputation was the only solution.

We held the gerbil on Carolyn's cutting board at the kitchen sink. I carefully administered a small dose of ether anesthetic I had liberated from a friend's research lab. I retracted the tail skin about an inch and then snipped off the bone with Carolyn's sewing scissors. When I pulled the skin back down, it covered the remaining bone nicely. A few sutures in the skin with Carolyn's sewing needle and thread completed the procedure.

"Let's not mentioned this to Mama," I suggested.

It took Carolyn only minutes to detect traces of gerbil blood on the cutting board, the sink, and the scissors. She was not pleased.

The gerbil survived, and seemed never to have missed the tuft on his tail. The hamster survived despite indifferent care. Bill changed the shavings in the cage much too infrequently, resulting in a chronically smelly cage. Eventually, we moved the cage to a half bath just off the door to the garage.

The first wintertime cold front brought with it a freezing night. The next morning, there the hamster lay, stiff and cold on the floor of his cage. It was a sad day in the Fleet household. We delayed burial until late afternoon to allow me to go to work and the children to go to school. Carolyn lined a box with flannel, and I dug a hole in a flowerbed. We buried the hamster in his little coffin just at dark, and stood in a cold misty rain while Bill played a sad song on his flute. We had our closure. I was secretly glad. We had buried a nuisance.

That summer, I related the hamster story to my sister. Her children had kept gerbils, hamsters, mice, and other varmints.

My sister asked, "Was it unusually cold the night he died?"

"It sure was."

"That hamster wasn't dead. He was hibernating. Ours used to do that often."

I thought, "Well, he's dead now."

And then there were rabbits. Our children persuaded us to buy white rabbits as pets. We seemed never to learn. Undomesticated animals usually do not make good pets.

I built a wire pen and a small shelter for our two new animals. Unfortunately, one was male and one was female, and they began to reproduce like, well, rabbits. Before long, the pen contained six or more white bunnies. (It was impossible to get an accurate count because they had honeycombed the pen with tunnels, making it look like a World War I no man's land. I never could be sure how many bunnies were underground.)

One night, a neighbors' hound climbed into the pen. The next morning, the dog sat in the pen surrounded by dead rabbits. I know dogs cannot smile, but he seemed to be doing just that. I could tell he was extremely proud of his night's work.

I let the dog out, picked up the dead rabbits and, once again, felt more relief than grief.

The pen lay dormant, displaying not a single sign of life for three days. Then, as I left for work, I saw two long white ears protruding from one of the tunnels. They looked like a large, white, furry V. I doubt it was a victory sign. Perhaps it was a peace sign.

I thought, "Maybe I can borrow our neighbor's hound dog tonight."

Up and Down the Ductwork with Mop and Broom

Tic-tic-tic; tic-tic-tic penetrated into my consciousness. Wonder what's that noise? Maybe one of the neighbors is doing something outside. The noise persisted, punctuated by pauses of various lengths.

Nope. No activity in either neighbor's yard. What could that noise be? Sounds metallic, like scratching. Oh, no! Maybe a skunk or possum, or maybe a squirrel. Plenty of those varmints in our yard, and it's getting cooler. I bet whatever it is, it's trapped in the ductwork under the house.

The air conditioner company sent a man the next day. He found no obvious evidence of varmint invasion, but considerable insulation had been chewed off some of the ducts.

I asked, "What should I do now?"

"Let us clean the ductwork. If some animal is there, they will find it. We can replace the insulation while we're under there."

"Okay."

At eight o'clock a.m. on the scheduled day, a huge green truck pulled up to our back door. Three men alit and began preliminary preparations. I mentioned the likelihood of an animal. The company had neglected to make them aware of that possible complication. They did not seem happy.

I assumed skunk spraying was a likely possibility.

The three spent most of the morning manning air pressure hoses and brushes in the ducts. A twelve-inch diameter hose connected my ducts to their truck. The truck sported eight six-foot dust bags that protruded from the top like overgrown sausages—sort of a vacuum cleaner on steroids. After lunch, two other air conditioner men joined the original three. They blew and brushed and sucked until every duct had been cleaned. No varmints turned up, to everyone's profound relief.

A preliminary inspection under the house had revealed a small leak in a water heater. I called my plumber. He came over promptly, inspected it, and replaced it with a new one that afternoon while the air conditioner men worked inside the house.

In the midst of all the activity, both the lawn service and the house-cleaning services arrived. For part of the afternoon, my driveway and the street in front of the house contained two trucks from the air conditioner service, the plumber's pickup truck, the truck from the lawn service, the house-cleaner's van, my wife's car, and my pickup truck. One might have thought we were hosting a party with an eclectic guest list.

So, here I sit, totally exhausted even though all I did was watch. I have a new water heater, clean air ducts, a clean house, and a freshly mowed lawn. The ticking noise is gone. My bank account is significantly lighter.

I will relax and contemplate the joys of home ownership.

Backyard Bird Watching

I read a piece in the paper last week about the nationwide backyard bird survey this week. I thought I just might participate, since I have quite a number of birds that frequent my yard.

My house is almost in a wilderness. A creek lies along the back of our backyard. That is my wilderness: my thirty-foot-wide wild place, all grown up in brush and trees of all ages.

My wilderness makes a perfect haven for wildlife of all kinds. Squirrels love the treeline, and I can count over a dozen squirrel nests along our part of the creek. Our next-door neighbor waged a summer-long battle with squirrels in her backyard. She trapped one-hundred-and-sixty-seven and never made an obvious dent in the squirrel population. She released them about a mile away. I wonder if she had really trapped one-hundred-and-sixty-seven squirrels, or if she trapped the same squirrel one-hundred-and-sixty-seven times.

During our first winter in our new home, I heard loud rapping sounds emanating from the creek. Close observation revealed a huge woodpecker digging for insects in one of the tall dead trees along the creek bank. He was black, about a foot long, and had a prominent tuft of red feathers on his head.

I became curious about what kind of woodpecker stopped in my wilderness. I bought a book on bird identification and discovered that he was a Pileated Woodpecker. He or one of his relatives visited our creek every January for several years until the dead tree fell. I have never seen a Pileated Woodpecker since.

I soon became enamored of birdwatching. I acquired the common feeling that if I named a bird, I felt as though I owned him. I didn't need my book to name sparrows, robins, blue jays, doves, cardinals, goldfinches, and mockingbirds, and other birds very common in the South. I learned to name bluebirds and Ruby-Throated Hummingbirds and towhees and cowbirds and other, not-so-common birds. I learned not to call blackbirds "blackbirds," but to call them Purple-Headed Grackles though "blackbirds" still seems good enough for me. The differences between house finches and purple finches continue to baffle me. I never sought, nor saw, rare birds. Backyard birding was satisfying enough for me. But I fancied myself an expert in my niche.

One evening just at dusk, my wife and I drove into our backyard turnaround. As we opened the car door, we heard a rather loud, distinct hooting call.

Carolyn asked, "What was that?"

I replied, "Someone trying to imitate an owl. And not doing a very good job of it, either."

As we stepped out of our car, a very large Barred Owl silently flew from a nearby power pole.

Maybe I won't participate in the nationwide backyard bird count this year, after all.

Changing Needs

Our house may not be equal to the upscale million-dollar-plus houses boasted by others in the city of Brentwood, but we do have a room designed just for physical fitness.

We live in one of the original subdivisions of Brentwood, and like all of them in the subdivision, our house is over forty years old. There is nothing wrong with it. It is just dated. I tell my out-of-town friends we live in "Historic Brentwood."

The ceilings are eight feet; the living area is "chopped up" into distinct areas. Walls define a separate living-dining room, den, kitchen-breakfast room, and utility room. Our bonus room is up a few stairs and over the garage. Bedrooms, bathrooms, hall, and closets are smaller than rooms built today. In all, it is a good house and, like its owners, it has been around a few years.

About fifteen years ago, Carolyn and I decided the house needed a bit of upgrading, and began to plan. We decided to enlarge our master bedroom and bathroom and add new closet space. As floor plan drawings progressed, I pushed for a separate room for a treadmill. And so, we added a tiny room only four-and-a-half by nine feet. We installed a TV on a shelf in one end of the area, and a treadmill occupied the remainder of the space. This was our "workout room." Not up to Brentwood standards, but adequate for us.

Like people the world over, we started our aerobic work enthusiastically. It was not many days before the aerobic exercise began to pale. Even with the TV, it was so boring that it took what felt like an hour to do my thirty minutes' walk. I soon reverted to outdoor walks. At least I could see birds and trees and feel the breeze. An added advantage was that I could skip the walk in inclement weather without guilt. Carolyn walked bravely on.

Carolyn recently developed back problems requiring significant reduction in physical activities, including walking, and the treadmill evolved into what most home treadmills eventually become— expensive clothes hangers.

We gave the treadmill to our daughter, and wondered what to do with the odd little room opening into the bathroom—until I hit upon a solution.

We now have a four-by-nine library, equipped with shelves down one side and across the end—plenty of room to house our books, with some shelf space left available for later use. It contains almost all of my collection of over two hundred books I could not part with. They once occupied every horizontal surface in my walk-in closet.

I visit my library most every day, usually just to admire my collection, sometimes to pick out a book to reread or one for a grandchild to read. Home gyms are fine for the younger set, but a library has much more snob appeal. And there is always outside in good weather.

Crayfish and Cajuns

We lived only two hundred or so miles from northeast Louisiana—Cajun country. Daddy went down there almost every summer to buy cotton before the harvest began in our part of the country.

There was a custom in Cajun country: merchants drank a small cup of coffee with their customer after each transaction. Daddy told me of an old cotton trader who was so busy he drank about forty cups of coffee a day.

Daddy asked him, "Don't all that coffee keep you awake?"

He replied, "No, but it helps."

At least twice a year, Daddy brought home two bushels of live oysters in their shells. He always arrived home at night with ice enough to preserve the oysters at least until the next morning. Then the fun began.

We ate raw oysters on the half shell, and oysters Mama had fried and served hot and very crisp. Daddy forced me to down a raw oyster when I was six or so. I thank him for that every time I go into an oyster bar.

We had oyster stew, scalloped oysters, oyster dressing, oysters Rockefeller, oysters Bienville. Every way an oyster could be prepared, we had it.

And then he would bring home seventy-five or so pounds of crayfish, live of course. And we would have a crayfish boil. This is how we did it.

First they had to be purged. That's right, purged. I don't know why, but the experts said they did. We put the crayfish in a large vat filled with brine. After a few minutes, we drained the vat, refilled it with fresh water, drained that, and repeated the washing process two more times. Now we had pristinely clean crayfish, inside and out.

Then, they went into a large pot of boiling water containing corn on the cob and red potatoes. The corn and potatoes had been cooking while the crayfish purged. A short boil, and the crayfish were done. We poured off the water and dumped the food on a picnic table covered with several layers of newspaper. The cook sprinkled a liberal amount of Cajun spices over the entire pile.

We all sat around the table, dug into the pile, and extracted corn and potatoes and crayfish. Though not mandated by Emily Post, Jax Beer was mandatory if you drank beer. I always felt sorry for the non-beer drinkers.

We gnawed at the corn and popped pieces of potato in our mouths just enough not to be labeled a crayfish miser. Unlike shrimp that have two-thirds tail and one-third head, crayfish have the opposite, two-thirds head and one-third tail.

Daddy said many times, "Boiled crayfish give negative calories. It takes more calories to peel one than you get from eating one."

Real Cajuns didn't stop with the tails. They suck the juicy insides of the head and body. I only did that after my third bottle of beer.

Living as close to the Gulf of Mexico as we did, we had lots of seafood. Not only did we eat oysters and crayfish, but snapper and flounder and grouper and soft-shelled crabs often graced our table. Local catfish competed quite well with the more expensive Southern seafood selections. Rice and beans complemented dinners quite nicely.

We mostly ate chicken and pork and beef and rice and beans and vegetables from the garden. That fishy stuff was special. But indeed it was special, and is so even today. I know the next time I return home to Mississippi, we will have a crayfish boil.

And I will always think of Daddy at the crayfish table, and Mama at the stove frying oysters.

Food, Crime, and Sex

Stop the presses! (Or whatever one stops to add breaking news to an e-paper)

This just in: A local restaurant was robbed by a bearded man while his accomplice distracted the staff and customers by performing an exotic strip tease dance. The couple escaped without pursuit in a white 2009 Lexus SUV which blended into the dozens of upscale luxury cars within the environs of the city. They also ran several red traffic lights and were said to have turned left illegally at least once, further disguising their non-Brentwood identity.

This notice is pure fabrication. My intrepid editor told me that crime and food draw the greatest number of readers, so I am almost guaranteed publication of this story. I added the beard and exotic dancer just for spice, and the traffic stuff because Brentwood traffic is one of my many pet peeves.

And now I need to fill the rest of my allotted space. The short piece below fulfills that need.

Why I Write

I belong to writers' groups at the Martin Senior Center here in Brentwood.

Our group has published three anthologies. In the latest one, in addition to our other submissions, we each were required to write a short piece about why we write. This is why I write:

The question "Why do you write?" reminds me of my interest in dogs. As an adolescent, I became fascinated with the question, "Why do dogs bark?"

I spent hours reading scientific papers by dog behavior specialists. I even read about a breed of European dogs bred to protect sheep from wolves. Those dogs do not bark at all. They live with their sheep, blend in with the herd, and are aggressive only toward predators. I also found a breed of dog from the Netherlands that was bred to lie on the roofs of canal boats and bark aggressively at each approaching stranger to alert the owners of possible intruders.

Those are special breeds bred to bark or not to bark. But what about other breeds and what about mutts? Why do they bark? I did not have a clue.

Finally, I asked a kennel owner his opinion. He replied, "To tell you the truth, I think they bark just for the fun of it."

Why do I write? To tell you the truth, I write just for the fun of it.

Okra

I like okra. I like to grow it. I like to eat it. I like it fried. I like it boiled. I just like okra.

If you can't grow okra, you can't grow anything. It is a tropical plant, a relative of hibiscus and of cotton. These plants love the heat—the hotter the better. Okra needs only a modicum of water, and can grow in minimally fertile soil. It bears from late spring until the first significant frost in the fall. I have never heard of an okra crop failure.

Many people don't like boiled okra because they claim it is slimy. It won't be, if you pick it when the pods are finger-sized and if you leave the little tam cap on during cooking (left on the okra, not the cook). It goes great with homegrown peas and homegrown beans.

Fried okra is a real delicacy. Not the kind served in restaurants or available pre-breaded in the store. That okra is mostly breading, and tastes that way. Gourmet fried okra is merely covered with cornmeal and fried. Maybe a little salt and pepper can be added, if the cook desires. Original recipes called for bacon grease to fry it in. Modern cooks use vegetable oil. I suppose super health-minded cooks could use olive oil. I have never tasted okra cooked that way, but I just might try it someday if conditions are right.

Carolyn cooks healthily. She seldom, if ever, fries foods, so I seldom have home-cooked, real fried okra. But I once did.

Years ago, when Carolyn's mother had become too old to live alone, she hired a live-in companion. Understandably, the companion needed a weekly day away. Carolyn filled in for the companion for twenty-four hours every Wednesday. That day coincided with our weekly house-cleaning service, and also with one of my evenings free of night responsibilities. Since I was on my own for supper, it became my habit to pick okra from my garden, cut it up, cover it with cornmeal, and fry it as part of my supper.

Carolyn complained about the quality of the cleaning service. She was especially critical of the job they did in the kitchen. "They never clean the stovetop. It's always greasy," she said.

I kept quiet, hoping the storm might blow over. The next week, I cleaned the stovetop carefully. On Thursday, Carolyn complained about the stove again. The stove had never been so clean as after my scrubbing the next Wednesday, but it still failed to measure up to Carolyn's standards.

"I think I'm just going to hire another cleaning service," she said.

"I'll talk to them this week. Give them one more chance."

My days as okra chef were gone forever.

Gumbo

Seafood gumbo and crayfish etouffee are the pinnacles of gastronomic delight, at least for me. Nothing approaches their delicate aromas, their complex tastes, their textures. I cannot exist without real gumbo or real etouffee at least once a year. To omit my seafood stew fix for a year would undoubtedly be fatal.

I fell in love with my Middle-Tennessean wife-to-be, Carolyn, when I was in medical school. She had never heard of gumbo or etouffee and would not eat oysters. Gumbo is no mystery to Deep South housewives. I reasoned that Carolyn could at least learn how to make gumbo. My sister had a rather simple recipe that she shared with Carolyn. It contains shrimp, tomatoes, tomato paste, beef stock, and a little beef. Of course, okra is included along with celery, onions, bay leaves, thyme, garlic, Tabasco sauce, parsley, filé, and Cajun Creole seasoning—a very simple recipe. It does not include a roux, making it even simpler to prepare. I hate the strong-tasting sausage in some gumbos because it overwhelms the seafood flavors, so we leave sausage out.

Carolyn dutifully and carefully prepares the recipe once a year. (I guess she wants to keep her husband alive.)

One winter, we had some crabs in the freezer. "Put them in the gumbo," I suggested.

"But they're not in the recipe."

"Throw them in anyway."

She did, and we have included crabmeat and clams each year since. After all, gumbo evolved as a stew made with okra, filé, roux, and whatever seafood and vegetables that were available to a poor Cajun family.

Christmas night has become our traditional time for gumbo—for our entire thirty-person Middle Tennessee extended family. Carolyn and I cook about three gallons of the stuff. Forget country ham and turkey. Gumbo beats them both, hands down.

We start the gumbo about three days ahead of time. I cut up celery, onions, and garlic and Carolyn prepares beef stock. The day before Christmas, I peel ten pounds of shrimp, and Carolyn begins to cook. She puts the beef stock in a huge pot, adds tomatoes, tomato paste, a little beef, bay leaves, thyme, garlic, Tabasco, parsley, Cajun Creole seasoning, and the diced vegetables plus okra grown in our garden the previous summer. The mixture simmers all afternoon.

Finally, on Christmas Day, we add shrimp, clams, and crabmeat early in the afternoon, to cook until suppertime.

Christmas supper consists of gumbo served over steamed rice and with fresh French bread—nothing else.

Gumbo and French bread are a grand way to finish a full and exciting Christmas day.

Addendum:

With all the oil troubles in the Gulf, I may have eaten my last gumbo. Watch for me in the obits.

Chapter Eight, Hobbies and Pastimes

I lead a busy life, but I seldom get much done. My vegetable garden keeps me busy for most mornings in spring and summer. Fall and winter sees me in my woodshop making a variety of simple projects. At one time, I made simple furniture, but as I have grown older, I mostly make birdhouses and such.

Tools

Everyone has tools. I just happen to have a few more than most. Of course, I have yard and garden tools, too, but mostly I have woodworking tools.

I have a hand drill, a handsaw, a plane, and a drawknife that I bought sixty years ago. As soon as I could afford it, whenever I needed a certain tool to complete a project, I bought it.

About twenty years ago, Carolyn needed a narrow clothes-hamper for the hall outside our laundry room. She had searched unsuccessfully all over town for one of the proper size. Not only could she not find the right size, but complained that none sold for less than thirty-five dollars.

"I'll make you one," I volunteered. She accepted. I designed a Colonial-styled hamper, purchased materials, and set to work.

I found that, even with repeated adjustments, I could not saw boards square with my old, cheap table saw. It was worn out. Fortunately, Sears had contractor-quality table saws on sale, so I hurried off that very day. Sears had a six-inch jointer on sale, as well, and I came home with both tools—a seven-hundred-and-fifty-dollar bargain.

Carolyn never said a word. She just hung a red seven-hundred-and-fifty-dollar furniture-store price tag on her new hamper.

I have five hammers. Why do I need five when I have only two hands? I have a hammer for rough work, a hammer for finishing work, and a lightweight hammer to drive small nails. The other two are lightweight hammers for use by grandchildren.

In addition to my sixty-year-old hand drill, I own seven power drills and an additional hand-powered push-drill. An eighth-inch drill, two quarter-inch drills, a three-eighth-inch drill, a cordless three-eighth-inch drill, a half-inch drill, and a drill press are in my inventory. Each has its uses, though one quarter-inch drill I haven't used in years because it is worn out and virtually useless. I just can't throw away my forty-year-old, first power drill.

A partial list of my other hand tools includes twelve screwdrivers of various sizes, thirty-four clamps, eighteen carving chisels, eight pairs of pliers, four adjustable wrenches, a set of box wrenches, a set of socket wrenches, two hot-glue guns, two try-squares, a framing square, and six measuring tapes and rulers.

For finishing work, I can choose among four hand-held power sanders, two bench sanders, and two routers.

Then come the biggies: standalone power tools. I have a radial arm saw and a thickness planer that I bought from widows of woodworker friends of mine. I used admirable restraint in waiting until the grieving widows had returned home from the cemetery before making my offers. Other big tools include a table saw, a band saw, a scroll saw, a jointer, and a lathe.

If it is made of wood, I can make it, though often with less-than-professional skill. I built a blanket chest for my son's fiancé several years ago. I had worked on it for weeks, and proudly showed it to one of my expert woodworker friends.

He looked at it intently from all angles and pronounced, "You hide your mistakes very well."

So, what do I make now? Things that do not require great skill, and nothing remotely useful. Although I have made simple furniture and hobbyhorses in the past, now I only make children's toys, bird feeders, birdhouses, and other low-stress projects.

Mostly I just make sawdust.

Higgins Boats

I once owned half a Higgins boat. But not the kind you might think.

The recent memorials to D-Day brought my Higgins boat to mind. You may have seen movie clips of landings from clunky little boats, each open to the elements with a square bow. You may have seen, innumerable times, the grounding on the beaches, the dropping down of that bow to make a ramp, and then tightly packed soldiers pouring off the boat, down the ramp onto the beach. Those boats were called "Higgins boats" because they were made by the Higgins boat company of New Orleans, Louisiana.

Their boats were derived from square-bowed work boats designed to be used in the oil fields. They were shallow draft with a bow that made a ramp, and as such, were quite versatile. One unusual feature was their construction. They were made of molded plywood. Each ply was molded over a master mold, layer by layer, to yield a strong, smoothly contoured shell.

Our Higgins boat had no resemblance to a landing craft. It had a sharp prow; had no room for more than two people; was only twelve feet long. Its only feature in common with the wartime boats that it was made of molded plywood. It was one of the Higgins Company's first post-war products.

My good buddy Bob and I fished often together, usually from the banks of ponds or from boat storage docks. I mentioned to Bob more than once how I wished for a fishing boat.

Bob said one day, "My father-in-law had a fishing boat, and it has sat in my mother-in-law's carport for years. He died quite a few years ago, and the boat has not been in the water since."

I lost little time inspecting the boat. It sat in a carport filled with newspapers. Its paint was faded and peeling. There were a few gouges along the rub rail, but the hull seemed otherwise intact. I carefully examined the boat for signs of rot and found none. I discovered a brass plaque in the bow stating that it was a Higgins boat, built in 1947.

I couldn't believe my good fortune. A genuine Higgins boat, made soon after WWII with the same molded plywood technique of the famous landing craft. I had to have that boat. I made a deal with Bob. I would repair any dings, repaint the boat inside and out, and replace the trailer and outboard motor. We could share equally in ownership. He took my deal.

We spent the winter scraping and sanding and painting. I made short work of repairing the few dings with mahogany inserts. By spring, we had a boat that looked and felt new.

After two fishing seasons, it became obvious our tiny boat was unsuited to the large TVA lakes of Middle Tennessee. We needed something more seaworthy. I bought Bob's share of the boat and struck a deal with a local boatyard for a new aluminum boat with all the accessories fishermen need (or want).

As I trailed the Higgins boat to the dealer, I noticed a car following me. He even followed me into the boatyard.

He asked, "Isn't that a Higgins boat? I have a big collection of Higgins boats and would love to have this one."

It was too bad, but he had missed his boat.

The dealer failed to appreciate what a treasure sat rotting on his yard. The little Higgins boat sat in the dealer's yard for two years, filled with rainwater, and quickly deteriorated into a pile of rotten wood.

I wish I had kept that boat.

Turnings

A few weeks ago, I saw a picture in the Tennessean showing a gaggle of Brentwood political bigwigs wielding shiny shovels. They were ceremoniously turning over the first earth in a construction project, a park, as I recall. They were posed in front of several posts and what appeared to be a table leg. The caption said the table leg was a corner post, but I have never seen wooden outdoor fenceposts sporting beads and coves. It obviously had been turned on a lathe—rather fancy for a fencepost. The corner posts in my yard might have been turned as well, if I had thought to do it years ago.

I really like to turn things on my lathe. The rapid change in shape of round stock into a decorative piece or making a goblet or a bowl from a large square of wood is great fun. The shape changes in front of my eyes, much like the immediate changes seen in shaping pottery. I wonder how long it would take me to turn a two-by-four into a toothpick.

I don't claim to be an expert woodturner. I am, at best, an accomplished beginner, whatever that is. I have turned goblets and bowls and drawer knobs, to name a few things. I think round balls are the hardest—more like impossible—for me to do a decent job on. The ball on top of my mailbox post is my best effort.

When I installed my croquet course, I needed a regulation-sized center post. It had to be eighteen inches tall and one inch in diameter. There was a post listed in my croquet supply catalogue listed for thirty dollars.

I thought, I can make my own post for almost nothing. I glued up some surplus oak flooring as my blank. It was easy to turn the post—just a cylinder. I added indentations to separate the four-color bands, added a sharpened end to drive into the ground, and rounded the edges of the top.

I needed to paint the post in regulation colors—basic white with red, blue, yellow, and black bands. I didn't have the proper colors for my bands, so I bought four small cans of enamel. The final cost of my homemade post was twenty-seven dollars—but I had fun making it.

One of my more ambitious projects was turning four finials to replace the ones lost from an antique four-poster bed. I designed the finials to harmonize with the posts, and set to work. The first finial was easy. Making three exact copies was much more difficult. Using the first finial as a pattern, I measured and marked and set calipers to the same depth of the coves as the original.

The first try at finial number two resulted in coves too deep. The second try was discarded when I let the chisel slip and dug a deep hole into a bead. After another mistake or two, I had four finials more or less alike. An hour's job had turned into an all-afternoon project, typical of my woodworking efforts.

When I delivered them to my friend I said, "Your new finials are not quite identical, but they do show a strong family resemblance."

Weeds

Botanists define weeds as unwanted plants, or plants growing where they are not supposed to be. I define weeds as pure nuisances.

It seems that weeds grow when nothing else can or will. My lawn was full of weeds last summer. But I let them be. If I killed the weeds, I would have a brown, bare ground—no lawn at all.

My garden was a near-total failure last year. Even with regular watering and fertilizer, I picked only a few squash, almost no zucchini, a smattering of peas, and absolutely no tomatoes. The only thing in my garden that thrived was my okra and, of course, weeds. I had a bumper crop of weeds—lots of crabgrass, Bermuda grass, and other plant pests I have no name for.

Despite hoeing and occasional herbicide applications, my weeds thrived. They seem to do that every year despite my best efforts. Nothing I do ever completely eliminates those pesky plants. I think the only solution for weeds is for some bright botanist to discover a commercially profitable use for weeds. Then our cultivated weeds would develop a myriad of blights and scales. Despite watering and feeding and careful pampering, the weeds would refuse to thrive.

Our weed patches would probably be taken over by nuisance plants such as beans and peas and squash.

Requiem for a Zucchini

Hot sun glares,
Consuming all it touches.
The grass,
The garden.
Cicadas sing
A song of love.
Without a mate, their line is dead.
Flowers droop.
Weeds grow tough.
Dogs lie panting in the shade.
The sun is hot,
Cicadas loud.
August presses down
As I'm picking black-eyed peas.

I wrote this little poem some three years ago after the record-breaking summer heat. It seems appropriate today. After the unusually severe winter we are in the midst of one of the hottest summer in years. (While I write this, a heat advisory is being reported on the TV news.)

If flowers had tongues, they would be holding them out today. My poor vegetables are worse. Squash is valiantly fighting and producing a few fruits; zucchini has given up; pea harvest is off; blackberries have quit after only six quarts of berries. Only okra is producing. But then, it is a tropical plant and thrives in heat. Squirrels have eaten every one of my tomatoes. The vines are soon to go. I'll plant turnip greens there next month. I didn't plant cucumbers or green beans this year. If I had, I doubt they would have been worth the trouble.

So here I sit bemoaning my fate and considering giving up the garden. I am defeated by the weather and the varmints. And yet, I have hopes for my turnip greens. Surely they will produce. They haven't failed me yet. Maybe the weather will moderate by then.

The heat and the inevitable infirmities of age have conspired against me this year. But all in all, I do like having seasons. And as a Vanderbilt graduate (twice) I have learned to chant, "Wait'll next year."

Why doesn't someone discover how to limit global warming to wintertime?

What Would Jesus Do?

I grow blackberries. I propagated the vines from a single plant, a gift from a nephew. Eventually, I had vines enough to produce about ten gallons of fresh berries every summer. That was about three times the amount we could eat, give away, or freeze. The leftovers eventually went into blackberry syrup. Lately, I have limited my vines to yield enough for two gallons for me, plus a feast for the birds.

Blueberries are a different kettle of fruit. Several years ago, I responded to an offer in a seed catalog and ordered several dwarf blueberry plants. I reasoned that dwarf plants should be unlikely to fight the blackberries for growing space in my garden. I ordered six plants, and set them out about three feet apart.

All my plants survived transplanting, though they seemed slow to produce new growth early in the summer. I attributed this delay in new growth to transplant shock, whatever that is. I fertilized and mulched the plants and hovered over the plants like a doting father. There was little new for the doting father to see that first summer.

The second summer seemed much the same. The plants grew very slowly, and produced only a few blooms. If they bore a few berries, birds got to them before I could. I fertilized and mulched again, and made certain the plants never suffered from a lack of water.

Third summer, same result. Maybe a handful of berries, too few to satisfy a bird—and none for me.

That autumn, our pastor preached a sermon from the parable of the farmer and his fig tree that refused to bear fruit. He decided to cut it down. His servant convinced the farmer to let him fertilize and mulch the tree once more, and cut it down the next summer if it did not bear fruit.

That afternoon I stood before my blueberry bushes and said, "You've had your chance. Not even Jesus would put up with you anymore." I cut the plants down and threw them onto the compost pile.

Backyard Battleground

Call me Mr. McGregor. I am a gardener. I usually grow blackberries, tomatoes, okra, corn, beans, peppers, cucumbers, squash and peas in my garden.

And my yard abounds with wildlife. It teems with squirrels, rabbits and chipmunks. Rabbits love the tender leaves of emerging okra, peas and corn and grow fat from my young plants. Unlike Mr. McGregor, my solution is tea. I make it from habanera peppers—the world's hottest, forty times hotter than jalapeños. The night after I spray the pepper tea, I often hear rabbits begging for water to ease the pain of their burning lips and tongues. To their timid tap, tap, tapings at my door, I answer, "Nevermore."

Our favorite garden vegetables are tomatoes, and the squirrels' favorite as well. Just as I do, they wait until tomatoes are at their reddest and juiciest before they eat. They take just a bite or two from each ripe tomato and then move on to the next. I could coexist with squirrels if they ate just one tomato at a time but too many squirrel-spoiled tomatoes hang from my vines. Something had to be done. Finally, I found that placing socks on the ripening tomatoes masked the color of the fruit, confusing the tomato-loving little buggers. What squirrel has ever heard of a ripe white tomato? It is so satisfying to outwit a squirrel.

Because of the rainy spring this year, I planted sweet corn in muddy rows, just poking seed into the ground. The next morning I found a neat little hole at every place a seed had been. Chipmunks! They had dug up every seed!

A second effort yielded the same result. After the third planting, I sprayed each row with pepper tea. Chipmunks deserved a hotfoot from the way they have treated me. Same result and not a sore-footed chipmunk in sight.

I covered my fourth planting, some with fine-mesh hardware cloth and some with plastic. The next morning I discovered holes in the plastic and tunnels under the hardware cloth.

I set a Haveaheart trap and baited it with peanuts. I haven't caught a single chipmunk, even though I shelled the uncooked nuts for them. Seed corn performed no better. It's not only butterflies that are free.

I am on the road to total defeat. Unless I can think of something else to do, I risk a major garden disaster. But what can I do? The mighty chipmunk owns the night.

The Great White Hunter

We love the creek that runs along the rear of our lot. It gives us the feeling of living in a rural area, though our wilderness is no more than thirty feet wide. Thirty feet is wide enough to harbor many squirrels and a variety of songbirds. We see turkeys and deer occasionally, as well. I welcome all this wildlife, but draw the line at skunks. A person can be just so tolerant and no more.

Our bird feeders provide rations for squirrels as well as birds. Unfortunately, they also feed skunks. Although I have no studies to support my contention, I think skunks seem to prefer sunflower seeds above almost any other food.

After a week of lingering skunk odor in our yard one spring, I called the Critter Ridder man who brings a trap and charges fifty-dollars whether or not he catches anything. He caught a possum and nothing else during his trap's stay.

My hardware store close by had a going-out-of-business sale and I acquired a large Haveaheart trap for half price. I carefully baited the trap with a sardine and placed it near our shed. I checked the trap from a safe distance that afternoon and could see a large black-and-white animal in the trap.

I ran to the house and shouted, "Who said skunks are nocturnal? I caught one today in broad daylight!"

Carolyn said, "The neighbors have a black-and-white cat."

Surely it wasn't the cat. Surely not! The cat wouldn't dare! I approached the trap very, very cautiously, and eventually opened the trap. The maddest cat in the city of Brentwood made a black-and-white blur across our yard on his way home.

I switched bait to sunflower seeds and caught no more cats. I did reduce the skunk population by eight that summer.

Homecoming at Eagleville

Norman Rockwell would have loved it! A snapshot of rural Americana. The very first Eagleville High School Fall Homecoming celebration.

It was one of those once-a-year days when the first autumnal cold front brings cool, high cloudless skies, a gentle north breeze, and an unbelievably bright, clear atmosphere that seems to sparkle like light flashing from a well-cut diamond.

We arrived thirty minutes early, and at the edge of town encountered the junior member of the two-man Eagleville police force, a Barney Fife with a loaded gun. Barney directed us to a parking space on Main Street far from the center of activities, and we accepted the place without argument. No one messes with Eagleville's Barney Fife!

At least five hundred locals lined the route, many sitting on dropped-down pickup tailgates and others sitting in lawn chairs. Tailgaters tended toward blue denim overalls. Behind us, at Joyce's Beauty Shack, women wearing plastic capes with hair in rollers or tied with strips of aluminum foil stood on her porch where they could see the parade and wave to the participants, all of whom they knew.

Promptly at one p.m. the parade began. We heard drumbeats and soon saw the Eagleville Marching Twenty, dressed in their bright new uniforms marching smartly to the drummers' cadence, doing their best to imitate the Corps of Cadets at West Point. This was the first year for a marching band, as well as football team, and they were not yet able to play well while marching. Twelve uniformed cheerleaders followed the band.

Then came the floats. Every class, kindergarten through twelfth grade, was represented. Since the Huntland Hornets were the visiting team, every float featured some mayhem to be inflicted upon hornets. Hornets were swatted, sprayed, splattered, and nailed. All floats rode on large flatbed trailers pulled by pickup trucks, and several of the float-riders held up a single finger and shouted, "We're number one," despite Eagleville's winless record.

Kindergarteners lead the procession. Thirty five-year-olds sat on their float, dressed in pith helmets and large grocery bags cut to resemble hunting jackets. They were on safari, waving large paper flyswatters at a giant paper-maché hornet emerging from an enormous paper- maché nest. That my granddaughter was one of the swatter-wielders did not at all influence my judgment placing her float as the best one in the parade.

At the rear of the parade came open convertibles carrying first the middle-school queen and her court, and next, the high-school queen and her attendants. All the high-school royalty wore similar long, white, backless dresses. Is "backless" the latest style?

Once the parade was finished, it was off to the new football stadium for the presentation of the high-school queen and her attendants. (My grandson escorted one of the attendants. I do not understand why he did not escort the queen.)

Finally, the winners of the float competition were announced. The kindergarten won in the elementary division, and rightfully so, but was edged out of the grand championship by the ninth-grade float, a miscarriage of justice to my mind.

The game started at seven o'clock, and Eagleville lost thirty-five to thirteen, but my grandson scored both of Eagleville's touchdowns. It was a good day. Anna's float won, and Jesse played well. Being grandparents can be great fun, and despite television and the Internet, small-town rural America still lives, little changed from the way it was fifty years ago.

Addendum:

The last game of the season was "Senior Night". Jesse was one of the seniors.

They won! Thirty-eight to seven. Their first win ever! They must be the only team in Tennessee that had a successful season with a record of one and nine.

Football

High football season is upon us. Grudge games are the norm. Warm up games are mostly over. Sports pages are full of football. Game schedules take up half a page. I can watch games for three nights a week and all day on Saturdays and Sundays. And some games are even exciting. I like football season.

Recently, stories have appeared on TV and the paper about college conference realignments. Conferences are losing teams and adding teams at a pace I have never seen before. Our conference, the Southeastern (SEC), has invited two new teams to join making the SEC a fourteen-team conference. For decades, the SEC had ten teams, until a few years ago when Arkansas and South Carolina joined.

Until now, we had a tidy little conference based on geography. All teams were in the southeastern part of the country. The addition of Texas A&M violates the concept of eastern, and the University of Missouri strains the integrity of south—at least in my mind. I have always considered Missouri as a border state. I hope accepting the school into the SEC doesn't rekindle the guerilla warfare of the Civil War one-hundred-and-fifty years ago. Surely those hostilities have cooled a bit by now. And surely there is enough hostility among the present states with Tennessee-Florida, Tennessee-Alabama, Auburn-Alabama, Florida-Georgia, and Ole Miss-Mississippi State yearly battles.

You may note the absence of Vanderbilt and Kentucky football teams from the list above. They seldom win in the SEC. We have to wait for basketball for that.

Not only is the SEC changing, but it seems that almost all conferences are realigning this year—some as a result of losing teams, and others hoping to cash in on that big pile of money from television rights. With all the realignments, conference names mean less and less. For several years the Big Ten (formerly the country's premier football conference) has had twelve members. The Big East is flirting with adding SMU, Houston, and Central Florida for a conference that will hardly be pure east anymore; the Big Twelve plans to shrink its membership back to ten when Missouri leaves. I don't know what other teams left or when they did, but it seems odd to me to retain the name Big Twelve with only ten teams.

Other conferences with geographic designations (like the SEC) are adding teams that render the conference names suspect. If the Big East adds SMU or Houston (both Texas teams) they will no longer be purely east. The Pacific Ten is now the PAC 12—and Arizona, Utah, and Colorado have very little ocean frontage.

Schools are looking for a TV bonanza, and old rivalries and loyalties are taking a backseat to big money. I can hardly blame them. Football is a big time, costly enterprise with a big time payout thanks to TV. Big money is irresistible. But we should think about new conference names. I suggest we rename our conference, the SEC. It will no longer be undiluted southern nor pure eastern. Maybe we should call it the Grape Nuts Conference—after the cereal that is neither grapes nor nuts.

Colors

Not only are we the buckle of the Bible Belt, but Tennessee can be called the lacings of the football belt. Football dominates the South every autumn. We are inundated by flying balls kicked or thrown by (mostly) males from age ten to sometimes mid-thirties. To say we live and breathe football this time of year is a true but well-worn cliché.

Team logos abound and are widely displayed. Stadiums are crammed with spectators in home team colors (except at Vandy games). It is quite a sight to see a hundred thousand rabid fans in orange wildly cheering at UT games. I even know of a guy who wears orange underwear on Tennessee game days.

And almost every party given from August to February, perhaps with the exception of most wedding receptions, guests are encouraged to "wear your colors." Families gather around the Thanksgiving feast often dressed in orange or gold or blue or red or some other team color and give thanks not only for their food and health, but for good won-lost records as well.

I don't know if my family is different from the mainstream, but we are grads of a variety of institutions of higher learning. My wife attended UT for a year but transferred to Vanderbilt School of Nursing midway in her college career. I hold two degrees from Vandy as well.

My children hold degrees from University of North Carolina (3), University of Georgia, Western Kentucky, and the University of Louisville. Grandchildren have degrees or are working toward degrees at the University of Georgia (2), Georgia Tech, the University of Kentucky, Middle Tennessee State, Clemson, and Calvin College. A few nieces and nephews graduated from Ole Miss, Mississippi State, and Middle Tennessee State. Of course, there are dozens of in-laws, nieces and nephews with UT credentials, too.

So, how do we dress at family functions in the fall? In anything except school colors. Like discussions of politics and religion, school colors are banned at family functions at our house.

Bowl Games

Bowl season is finally over. Don't fret if you missed games in the first week or two. Most were real yawners. There were thirty-five games on TV over three weeks beginning December eighteenth. I had my fill by the time the BCS championship match between Auburn and Oregon was over on January tenth. Some games were a boring waste of time. Other games were exciting contests between outstanding teams. The BCS championship game between Auburn and University of Oregon was certainly all anyone would wish—unless you were an Oregon fan.

There have been bowl games as long as I can remember, and that is a long time. The first bowl game I remember was when I was about eight. I remember lying on the living room floor in front of the radio listening to the Rose Bowl. I don't remember who won, or even who played, but I remember listening with my parents, aunt, uncle, and cousins. (This was a time when television was experimental and limited only to a few places. I had never even heard of it.)

Until several years ago, bowl games were limited to the Sugar Bowl, Cotton Bowl in early afternoon on New Year's Day, the Rose Bowl in late afternoon, and Orange Bowl that night—four games between eight outstanding teams in one marathon day. Sometime later, the Gator Bowl was added about a week before the others. Even at that time, television broadcasts were available only in the larger cities in the South so I had to settle for radio when Vanderbilt played in its lone Gator Bowl appearance.

Now, television, seems to rule sports. They have the money to call the tune, and bowls have multiplied like chipmunks in my garden. In addition to the traditional five bowls and the BCS championship bowl, we have a wide variety of lesser bowls.

There are concept bowls: the Independence Bowl, the Fight Hunger Bowl, the Humanitarian Bowl, and the Holiday Bowl.

There are geographic bowls: the New Mexico Bowl, the New Orleans Bowl, the Hawaii Bowl, the Alamo Bowl, the Texas Bowl, and of course, our very own Music City Bowl. I guess the state of Texas deserves two geographic bowls simply because of the size of the state.

And then there is the plethora of commercially named bowls: the Meineke Care Bowl, the Beef O'Brady Bowl, the Outback Bowl, the Little Caesar's Bowl, the Maaco Bowl, and the Chick-Fil-A Bowl. The sponsoring companies aim to stimulate our tastebuds and, of course, we can get our cars fixed if we have a problem on the way to one of the restaurants at half-time.

I really don't know where to fit in the BBA Bowl, the Pinstripe Bowl, or the Military Bowl into my concepts, but they were on the bowl schedule. And how about the GoDaddy.com Bowl?

Somehow I miss the one-day, four-game mini-marathon on New Year's Day. They all promised exciting games between top teams, and sometimes even delivered on that promise. Whether or not the games were exciting, they still represented contests between the best.

Contests between two 6-6 teams do little to stir my interest, but then, we fans seem to like our team in a bowl no matter how obscure the bowl may be. And I did become a bit excited at the Music City Bowl two years ago.

Athletics, Observations of a Casual Fan

Like most American men, I have followed sports all my life. I played most of the team games in high school—some better than others. I carried over that interest in sports to college—interest, not participation.

I have followed the vagaries of Vanderbilt intercollegiate sports for over fifty years—over good times and lean times. In my freshman year, 1951, the chancellor announced that football exerted too much influence on campus. He said it should be deemphasized to a level that fits in with the primary goal of the university: to educate students and contribute to the body of knowledge in the world. Deemphasization took. Vanderbilt football has never reached prominence it enjoyed a generation ago.

Despite their consistently losing ways, Carolyn and I attended most home games. Too often, the few years promising future improvement were followed by a return to mediocrity. It became too painful to watch their futility, and we gave up our season tickets several years ago.

Beginning in the early 1950s, basketball wagged the tail of Vanderbilt athletics. Coach Bob Polk dug the foundation, and Roy Skinner led teams always fighting for the SEC championship even though they usually finished second to Kentucky. The cry, "Wait for basketball," in football season rang out often and loudly. I particularly enjoyed watching Skinner's teams. They played fast-paced, high-scoring game best described as, "run, gun, and turn it over." Their philosophy seemed to be to let the other team shoot, grab the ball, fly down the court, and put it up. I remember Babe Taylor, the brother of one of my medical school classmates. He always seemed to race down the court dribbling at top speed while holding up one, two, or more fingers signifying an offensive play, then without pause, making a shot from the top of the key.

Sadly, the team began to struggle to maintain a place near the top of the league. Our season seats were moved from under the goal to the back row of the new balcony, and then a surcharge was added to our season ticket cost. Mediocre teams and a surcharge for the worst seats in the house proved too much. We gave up.

And now, things seem to be looking up. The basketball team has gone to the NCAA tournament for several years, and shows promise of success this year. The women's basketball team is a perennial conference power, and the baseball team reached the college world series last spring.

There seems to be a ray of hope for football, as well. They played with enthusiastic abandon this year, and next year's recruit class seems to be outstanding.

The only thing I see needed to cinch the new football fortunes is for them to be placed on probation for a year or two.

Television

As is my habit, I cut out and keep the football schedule from the Saturday morning paper. Fall is football time, and I spend most of every Saturday watching. There is a huge selection of games televised every week. I counted twenty-seven games on last week's schedule. The first games began at eleven a.m. and the last games started at nine-thirty p.m. We are offered so many choices that it is impossible to see every game every week. It was not so long ago that our choices of TV games were quite limited.

September twenty-ninth marked the sixty-first anniversary of the first live broadcast of a football game. There was only a single game broadcast that day, and I watched it—sort of. One of my father's business partners invited my father and me to see the telecast. The partner was one of those people who bought the biggest and newest of everything. He had the first television in town. There was no cable then, nor dish antennae. The signal had to be picked up through an external antenna. We lived over one hundred miles from Memphis, the nearest station to broadcast the video signal. Neither antennas built into TV sets nor rabbit ears were up to the job of such a long-distant reception. Only outdoor antennas would do. Because of the distance from the broadcasting station, the signal could only be received by an antenna some thirty feet high or higher. Since the signal was on the very edge of possible reception, atmospheric disturbances often disrupted the transmission of the signal, resulting in poor picture quality.

My dad and I arrived at his partner's house a bit late and were ushered into the TV room. It was lit only by the ten-inch, dimly glowing screen housed in a wooden console about the size of a kitchen stove. Several people sat raptly staring at ghostly-white figures moving about through myriads of white dots vibrating in a totally random pattern. It was far, far removed from watching actual players playing an actual game on an actual field. I could not even testify that there was a game being played. Sound reception was also poor.

We left in the second half to listen to the game on our radio at home. Football on TV has come a long way since that day.

Sailing

Sailing rivaled my love for flying. Like flying, I had no chance to pursue my infatuation during my childhood. My family couldn't afford a sailboat, and there was no body of water big enough for sailing within a one-hundred-mile radius. As a result, my sailing was limited to the design and construction of model boats. They were ungainly things that would stagger across the nearby bayou when the wind was gentle and the bayou was full.

When we were established in Nashville and finances allowed, I bought a used nineteen-foot open wooden sailboat. It had been well-maintained and the sails, though old, were quite serviceable. Except for my wife and children, the boat became my greatest love.

I refinished the hull inside and out, and repainted the trailer. I took several informal sailing lessons from its previous owner and began my career as the owner and captain of a fine yacht.

The first year or so after I had acquired the boat, I puttered around the lake, usually with my wife and my three children. Only my son, our oldest, shared my enthusiasm for sailing. Carolyn and the two girls endured. To Carolyn, wavelets lapping at the bow and the boat on a gentle heel meant her hair was being mussed and we could turn over at any minute.

One afternoon, Carolyn cried out when a gentle puff of wind suddenly increased the angle of heel, "Be careful. We might turn over."

I reassured her, "All skippers turn their boat over a time or two."

She said, "Turn over next week when I'm not with you and get it over with."

Not every outing was pure delight. Sitting in an open boat with the temperature of ninety and not a breath of wind is abject misery. Riding out a thunderstorm is pure terror. The howling wind and lightning flashes enforce the adage that says, "My boat is so small and the sea is so big." It is almost a certainty that the boat will capsize if one tries to sail through the storm, and the mast acts as a thirty-foot lightning rod.

One afternoon, Carolyn and I had sailed far from our dock when a thunderstorm boiled up and headed for us. There was no escape. I had proved more than once that sailboats cannot outrun storms. All we could do was to douse the sails and anchor, hoping the storm would veer away.

The storm passed with only a moderate wind and heavy rain. I noticed Carolyn crouched in the cockpit shivering and becoming wetter by the minute. I pulled the mainsail over her to shield her from the worst of the rain. When I did, about five gallons of water poured out of a fold in the sail directly onto her head.

She screamed, "What are you doing?!"

"I'm trying to help you."

"Don't try to help me ever again!"

That was Carolyn's last sail.

The Horse Show

It was Anna's first time in the ring. Our granddaughter competed in her first real horse show. This was not a Saturday casual show. It was the real thing, held at the Williamson County Ag Center over three days. It was the first one for Carolyn and me as well.

I thought horse shows would be a big improvement over dance recitals. At my first one of those, when our daughters were beginners, I planned to go early, see their pieces scheduled early in the program, and then slip out and go home. I was sadly mistaken. Dance teachers know all about reluctant fathers. They include every student in the finale— just to keep us at the recital.

We arrived at the Ag Center at about four o'clock, in plenty of time to park and to find Anna. We parked next to the barn between two large horse trailers, and stepped out into a sea of horses and riders and parents. All riders were dressed identically in black helmets, white shirts, black coats, tight tan pants, and black boots. An aura of pervasive, grinding tension from contestants and horses mingled with odors of horse droppings. Once riders mounted, tension seemed to ease somewhat, but still remained.

Classes entered the judging ring and were rated with practiced efficiency. Amazingly, all evidence of nervousness disappeared from each rider upon entering the judging ring.

When I was told that Anna would ride in one class Friday night and three on Saturday, I assumed they would be grouped early in the schedule, where beginners should be. Horse teachers must have taken lessons from dance teachers, because Anna rode once Friday night, once early Saturday afternoon, and then in two classes Saturday night, the last events of the evening. We got home Saturday night at ten. Mercifully, Sunday was reserved for Western riding.

Nine novice riders competed in the last two events. All young middle-school-age girls rode together to be judged on their horsemanship. Early in the competition, one horse bolted. He discarded his sedate trot and quickly threw his rider. A second horse then became agitated and unceremoniously dumped his rider on her head. Both riderless horses galloped around the ring dodging the other seven horses and eluding all attempts at capture. The judges quickly ordered the other riders to dismount and hold their horses beside the arena walls. It took at least fifteen minutes for eight adults to catch the runaways. Only when the horses tired did they submit to a hand on their bridles. Neither thrown rider appeared to be injured.

The remaining seven competitors and one of the thrown girls remounted and finished the event.

It was quite a spectacular finale. Much more exciting than a dance recital.

I wonder what next week's finale will be.

Chapter Nine, Wheels

Everyone has a car. It seems most of us are two-car families. Our American culture dictates those conditions. With three children two years apart, we had five cars for a number of years. My car was always the newest. It was essential for my medical practice that my car always could move at a moment's notice. Though those emergencies were infrequent, I had to have a dependable car.

Carolyn drove a stationwagon for over ten years during the time our children were in college. They drove an assortment of well-used hand-me-down vehicles, always subject to mechanical failure.

My First Half-Car

Almost nobody had a car at Vanderbilt during my undergraduate years in the early 1950s. I was among the majority, one of the withouts. By my last year in undergraduate school, my roommate, Gale, and I had girlfriends, but dating was difficult without transportation. The desire was there, but the wherewithal was not. We were in dire need of wheels. Style, color, make, and model were of only minor importance. After some serious searching, we became the proud joint owners of a jewel of a car, a 1942 black Chevrolet four-door sedan. The paint was dull; the seat covers were thin; the tires were suspect; there was no radio. But it met our major demand—cost.

The car had one obvious defect—the linkage between the gearshift lever and the transmission was broken. Gale's father repaired it with coat-hanger wire, but the repair was somewhat less than perfect. As a result, only he, Gale, and I could shift the car out of first gear. The gearshift problem turned out to be a tremendous benefit since no one could borrow our car. (The pressure on car-owners to loan their cars to friends was enormous.)

Our car had one other little problem—heat. The heater would not produce enough of it in the winter, and the radiator would not get rid of enough of it in the summer. If conditions were right, the windows would be covered with ice on their inner surfaces while the radiator steamed. Because we lost so much coolant through leaks and boiling overflows, we stopped buying antifreeze and just drained the radiator if sub-freezing weather was predicted. When I drove it home to Mississippi, I had to stop every one hundred miles or so to refill the radiator, once from a nearby creek. I had two passengers going home, but none going back.

After my admission to medical school, I sold my half-interest to Gale. He drove it for three years while earning his PhD in nuclear physics.

Even with its problems, the car was a godsend. It provided us with moderately dependable transportation and only minor inconveniences. And it improved our love lives immeasurably.

My Little Gray Truck

In anticipation of retirement, I decided to sell my car and buy a truck. That same year, 1997, my brother in law retired from farming and traded his truck for a car.

I read Consumer's Report and a magazine containing automotive pricing data. I chose the safest and most reliable small pickup, and knew to the penny how much I should pay. I spent an unhappy morning at one dealership haggling with a sales manager through a young salesman-go-between, and after a morning of very frustrated waiting, I stalked out. I would go somewhere else.

This time, I asked for and was introduced to an experienced salesman who had some clout. He toured me though their lot and, like a puppy in a pet shop, a gray extended-cab Ford Ranger jumped out, begging me to take it home. Nevermind that it lacked the cruise control that I had wanted, that truck had to be mine. I made my offer; the salesman left to talk with the sales manager, then returned in five minutes saying, "We have a deal. I told my boss that you were in no mood to haggle, and if we did, you would walk out." He was right.

I said a sad goodbye to my old Honda; a good car, but no match for a truck. I could haul big things in a truck, smelly things in a truck, and if I had a hitch and a trailer, I could pull a trailer with my truck. My first load was manure for my garden, and it was not long after I retired that I had a boat trailer and a hitch to fasten it to.

After seven years, the Ranger has been washed once and has acquired several dings, contributing to its personality. There are several dents in the license plate and tailgate from hits while hitching up my trailer. There are a long scratch on the right and a short scratch on the left from close encounters with a concrete post and a mailbox. A dent in the right rear fender perfectly matches the dent in the steel post supporting my grandsons' basketball goal. It lost a hubcap somewhere, too, and other dents and scratches have appeared out of thin air.

I have a bumper sticker that says, "Promote catfish. Run over a Chicken," but there are no bobblehead dolls, Saint Christopher's statues, or gun racks. But even so, my truck is still pretty much a guy thing.

Last year, I felt that I needed an SUV. I wanted to take more than one friend with me to go fishing, and it would be nice to have cruise control, an adjustable steering wheel, and power windows as well. An SUV could have all those things.

Once again, I poured over Consumer's Report and bought another automotive magazine. Then I began to think. I would have to sell my truck. It had so few miles on the odometer that a trade-in would cost me hundreds of dollars. But if I sold it privately, I would have to advertise it, ride along on test-drives, transfer the title, and buy new license plates. I would have to buy an expensive trailer hitch for my new SUV. I no longer would be able to walk down my truck bed onto the trailer tongue to board my boat with dry feet… not a big problem except in wintertime. Even worse, I would lose my bumper sticker.

New problems surfaced every day. Buying an SUV became a complicated process… a lot of trouble. Finally, it dawned on me. I did not want to give up my little gray truck. Instead, the truck and I had a heart-to-heart talk, and decided that we would just grow old together.

Scratches and Dings and Dents and Such

College tuitions and cars are more necessity than luxury in this society. That we had three children in four years complicated our finances during that period. Loans and a scholarship helped with tuitions. Cars were different. We solved that problem by hand-me-downs.

Our son, Bill inherited my old Malibu and passed it down to Cathy, our older daughter when he inherited a Dodge Dart from his grandfather. In time, all our children drove hand-me-down cars, each with its own problems.

Bill's Dart was unique among our stable of clunkers. His grandfather had driven it for four years and had neglected maintenance. It had several dents and scratches, and its finish had faded to a dull dirt color. The oil had never been changed.

Bill accepted his new car without complaint, and immediately set out to install a sound system appropriate for a college student. He bought an elaborate system, and spent all day installing it. The installation finally was successful after several modifications of the car, including permanent removal of the dash. He had the finest sound—in the junkiest car—on the campus.

He drove the car through college and most of medical school. During his senior year in college, it carried more students than it should to basketball games throughout the Southeast. The team was very good, his grades were very good, and the basketball odyssey was well deserved. They drove fast through the weekend nights with the car overloaded with boys. They named the car the "Death Dart." Fortunately, it never lived up to its name.

The car endured dings and scratches in campus parking lots, enough so that when one minor bump occurred, he could not identify the new one and he and the other driver parted ways without filing accident reports.

One accident was a bit more involved. He was stopped behind a car at a traffic light when a car slammed into him. The impact drove the Dart into the car ahead. Damage was significant, and a policeman was called. He spent time carefully documenting damages and assessing fault. Finally he approached the three drivers and said, "The car in front has major damage to his trunk lid and bumper. The car in back has destroyed his front bumper and grill. I can't find a single bit of damage to the car in the middle. It will make my report so much easier if we pretend the middle car didn't exist."

And that's what they did.

The Blue Malibu

Tuitions and transmissions kept us poor for years. Over a span of ten years, we financed eighteen college-years expenses and five decrepit cars. Our local mechanic had our telephone number on his hotline and we were on a first-name basis with financial-aid officers in five institutes of higher learning.

Bill, our oldest, inherited an old, dirty-brown-colored stationwagon from his mother as his first wheels. He drove his younger sisters to school every morning and hid the car in the far reaches of the school parking lot. An old, brown stationwagon is the epitome of uncool. When the stationwagon died, he inherited the blue Malibu, my work car that I had driven for three years—and it had been totally depreciated for income tax purposes. Shortly after he acquired his new blue wheels, Bill lost control trying to dodge a dog crossing the road and ran into a bridge abutment. A trip to the body shop for cosmetic surgery and straightening the bent frame restored the Malibu to a semblance of its former self.

Bill left for college,, and then 16-year-old Cathy inherited the Malibu. Her accidents happened in our driveway. A chronic dawdler, Cathy always left for school at least ten minutes later than she should. She would grab her books, race to the car, gun the car in reverse to turn around, and fly out of the drive toward school. One morning, I returned home in the pre-dawn from an emergency call and parked behind the Malibu. As was her routine, she gunned her car in reverse and BLAM, slammed into the rear quarter panel of my car. She threw the Malibu into drive and sped off toward school as though nothing had happened. She repeated the performance the first morning after Bill returned from college at Christmas break and had parked his hand-me-down Dodge Dart (a.k.a, the Death Dart) behind her. When Cathy entered college, she inherited my work car that she had backed into. At Christmas, our neighbor asked about the dent on the quarter-panel.

She replied, "Daddy did it."

Tricia was the fourth owner of the Malibu. Her first accident was a minor fender-bender in the school parking lot; not her fault, she claimed. It was not long until she had improved the quality of her accidents. While Carolyn and I were in Florida for an autumn vacation, Tricia, in violation of our strongest admonitions not to let anyone ride with her while we were away, drove her car down narrow Wilson Pike with the car filled with friends, and, distracted, ran off the road, bending sheet metal and the frame once again.

Within a year, she had turned too sharply into a Brentwood tack shop and ran off the end of a culvert into a deep ditch. This was the Malibu's last trip to the shop. Though only nine years old, it was declared to be a hazard to drive and pronounced dead. It was not the total mileage on the odometer that aged it so severely; it was the miles behind a tow truck that did it in.

Chapter Ten, Health

I consider myself to be healthy—at least as healthy as most of my contemporaries. I admit I don't exercise as much as I should, but only a very few men my age do. Even so, I have had my share of medical problems. I have survived coronary artery bypass, radical prostatectomy for cancer, cataract surgery, treatment for chronic bronchitis, and allergies—but I am basically healthy, at least in my own eyes.

Syncope

For weeks, Anna, my eighteen-month-old granddaughter, would point to a spot on our driveway and say, "Right there, right there. Granddaddy went night-night right there."

It had been only about six months since my radical prostatectomy for cancer, and my urinary continence was still a bit unreliable. I had tried to lessen the problem by limiting my fluid intake. I stayed thirsty all the time.

On a warm May afternoon, Carolyn, Anna, and I spent the afternoon visiting nurseries, buying plants for our deck and flower gardens. Just as I finished unloading the last flat, I fell to the concrete with a splat. Carolyn grabbed Anna, raced up the back steps and, with shaking fingers, dialed 9-1-1. As she frantically relayed the problem, our address, and other information to the emergency operator, I strolled into the kitchen.

"I'm going to kill you!" she screamed. "You have scared me and Anna almost to death." At my insistence, she canceled the EMT visit.

Sometimes it is not a good idea to have a cardiologist for a son. He found out about my little episode, came by our house on his way home from work, and stated firmly, "You have an appointment with my partner, Charlie Mays, tomorrow."

Tomorrow came all too soon. The initial physical exam revealed nothing unusual except that my blood pressure was only 90/60—rather low, and I wasn't even thirsty. The next day, I had an EKG, a stress test, a CAT scan, and a Doppler study of the blood flow in the arteries in my neck. All tests were normal.

The final conclusion was that I had become somewhat dehydrated that afternoon, which caused my blood pressure to drop even more. With the combination of low blood pressure, a very warm day, and more physical activity than I was accustomed to, I had simply fainted.

Just a simple case of not enough stress in my life.

Adventures Up and Down the Carotid Artery

Six days ago at seven a.m. (just after dawn it seemed), I introduced myself to a clerk at the hospital admitting desk. We exchanged pleasantries as she consulted her computer, pulled my papers, and fastened my ID bracelet to my arm.

Once again, I had a feeling of free-floating dread. With the acceptance of that bracelet I had surrendered every ounce of my independence. I was completely under the thumb of every doctor, nurse, orderly, and cook in this hospital. I must have felt somewhat the way one does when he is placed in jail. But my sentence was only two days, and there were no bars that I could see.

My cardiologist had kept an eye on my carotid arteries for at least ten years. Tests revealed slowly growing plaques in both arteries. Now the right carotid was about ninety percent closed, and complete obstruction could lead to a stroke. It was time to act, and here I was at the hospital starring in Act One.

I trailed a guide up two floors and down several halls to a room equipped with the usual hospital things. The dreaded hospital gown with two puny ties in the back lay neatly folded on the bed beside a plastic bag for my clothes. Slowly and reluctantly, I undressed, protesting all the while of the absurdity of taking off my undershorts for an operation on my neck. Protests fell on world-class deaf ears, and off came the shorts.

After a short wait, spiced by the inevitable vital signs and bloodletting, I was wheeled to the holding area. There I met my anesthesiologist and his trainee for a short review of my medical history, and for placement of a cannula in a vein and one in an artery.

I asked, "Why the arterial line?"

He replied, "It's routine in all vascular cases."

So, once again, I'm not someone special—just routine. I hoped I would remain routine— boringly routine. Good surgery is mostly boring. Excitement usually means complications.

They must have slipped something in my IV, because by the time I left for the OR, I was barely aware of what was happening. Once I was settled on the operating table, someone slapped a mask on my face and said, "I'm giving you a little oxygen." I was dimly aware of a not-unpleasant odor in the "oxygen," and awoke in the recovery room trying to get out of bed.

Eventually, I was moved to a room for the night. My pain was minimal, and I required no medications. I slept fitfully between visits by the nursing staff, and returned home in the early afternoon to finish my recovery.

I was impressed by the thoughtfulness of the entire hospital staff. They seemed genuinely concerned about my care and comfort. But I liked home better.

I have a scar from my jaw to my collar bone. Surgeons are fond of saying, "Wounds heal from side to side." But they hurt from end to end. They don't tell you that.

All in all, I prefer being a healthcare provider instead of a healthcare recipient—the sticker rather than the stickee.

Quality of Life

I scanned the news on the Internet this morning as I usually do. Side-by-side were short articles about the quality of life in various places in the United States. An article on the most stressful cities in the United States appeared adjacent to an article on the best places to retire in the United States.

There were five cities on the most stressful city list. Number five was Detroit. Crime and alcoholism were listed as problems there.

Jacksonville was fourth worst, according to this article. Crime and divorce rates were prominent.

Miami and suburbs ranked third. Again, crime and alcoholism were common.

Las Vegas was number two. Not surprisingly, crime and divorce rates were high.

Tampa-St. Petersburg was rated number one on the list. Suicides led the list. Other categories, while not leading, ranked high.

I was surprised that three of the top five stressful cities are in Florida. I always thought Florida was the place the older generation moved to retire—"to spend their Golden Years in uninterrupted pleasure." Maybe Florida is not the Eden I had thought.

The next article discussed the best places to retire. I have been retired for over thirteen years. Certainly I have experience enough to evaluate retirement living. The third best recommended retirement area was listed as "follow friends." Move to wherever your friends live. I can understand that. Living close to people with whom we have shared the highs and lows of our lives, and supported each other in trials and triumphs, is appealing.

The second recommended retirement site was to move near one's children. Being close to children and grandchildren is attractive. We can play with our grandchildren and get help from our grown children. I have several friends who have done just that—followed their children.

❧

The area receiving the highest recommendation as a retirement site is home—where one has lived longest, where roots are deep, where things are familiar, where we have old friends, and where we are comfortable. And that's just what we have done. We have stayed right here in Brentwood, in the same house we have lived in for thirty-seven years, going to the same church for forty-eight years, where most of our friends live, where two-thirds of our children and half of our grandchildren live, where it is described in the magazine, as one of the best places to live in the United States.

We were content to live here before the survey appeared. We see no reason to defy "expert" advice now.

And we own two cemetery lots.

Don't Call Me Elderly

Last week, the Brentwood Home Page issued a special notice from the Brentwood police warning us of a telephone scam present in our city. Residents received telephone calls congratulating them on their winning a hugely valuable prize. All the recipient had to do was to buy a five-hundred-dollar pay-as-you-go Visa card. The police emphasized that the scam targeted the elderly.

We were the recipients of three of these calls during the past week offering a "free" Mercedes. Both Carolyn and I turned the offers down out of hand, realizing the offers had all the markings of a con game.

I was proud that the Brentwood Home Page sent the message as a special extra item. I was not so proud to be referred to by the Brentwood police as "elderly." In fact, I felt a bit peeved. We are not elderly. We have no canes, no walkers, no home healthcare; do not live in a nursing home nor even in a retirement village.

It is true we pay to have someone to mow and to weed and prune the flower garden. My vegetable garden has only blackberry vines and three tomato plants this year, and my woodworking is limited to birdhouses, but the fertile soil and power tools are ready in case I feel the urge again. We don't use alarm clocks, and I only wear a tie on Sundays. I only write this column because it is fun.

I admit, we aren't as feisty as once we were. We don't run—nor even walk—as fast as once we did; we prefer matinees to nighttime plays and movies, but we can still stay up late if we need to. We still do things together, but attend more funerals than weddings. We share the same internist, the same dentist, and probably should have his-and-hers hearing aids.

We are mature. We aren't elderly.

What Do I Want To Leave When I Die?

I belong to two writers groups. In one, we merely read part of what we have written. I call it "Senior Show and Tell." In the other, we usually have an assignment for the next session. This column is one of the assignments I completed recently.

What do I wish to leave behind? That takes some thought.

First thought: money. Not much legacy from me. Our heir's money has been spent long since. We left the money to our children as tuitions, first cars, and down payments on houses. It was money well-spent. We still have enough money in our retirement account to support us for several years to come.

If not money, what? Forget the house. We plan to sell it in about three years and move into a retirement community. We have picked a first-class facility that will supply our every need. Its only drawback is that no children live there.

What about DNA? I have eight grandchildren who carry one-fourth of their DNA inherited from me. Every one of them is handsome, bright, and energetic. They each should make a positive mark upon the world and make their grandfather proud. That is a worthy legacy.

When I was younger, I planned to live hard and die young so that people viewing the body would say, "Doesn't he look good? Too bad he didn't finish his Great American Novel." I have outlasted those goals. It's hard to look good at seventy-seven, either dead or alive. And someone else will have to write my novel.

What would I really like to leave to the world? I think I would like to live so my epitaph can read, "He hath done what he could." (Mathew 14:8)

The Cycle of Time

I attend a writer's workshop twice a month at the Martin Center. Our facilitator suggests a topic for each session. We are encouraged (but not required) to write a short piece on the suggested topic. The last session's topic was "The Cycle of Time." I decided to write a poem with that as a theme. Though poetry almost never appears in this column, I decided to include this week's effort.

The Cycle of Time

Sunrise, Sunset, swiftly flow the days. Conceived only days ago, sees the light as new, breathes the air as new and cries.

Sunrise, Sunset, dressed in clothes all new and starchy. Pencil, crayons yet to mark. Alone, facing unknown foes. No mama to help.

Sunrise, Sunset, cap and gown, diploma, college challenges only days away.

Sunrise, Sunset, new cap, new gown, new paper in hand. Ready for the world.

Sunrise, Sunset, I-do's said a while ago. Someone to hold, someone to comfort.

Sunrise, Sunset, new life emerges into light, into air, cries.

Sunrise, Sunset, empty nest sometimes filled by baby's babies.

Sunrise, Sunset, doctor's bills and drugs, his-and-hers hearing aids.

Sunrise, sunset, swiftly flow the days

One season following another
Laden with happiness and tears.
(Inspired by the play, "Fiddler on the Roof")

Chapter 11, Miscellaneous

This final section contains twenty-five stories that I could not fit into any other logical category.

Close Encounters with Blue Lights

I guess we all have seen the dreaded blue lights in our rearview mirrors at one time or another. I am no exception.

My first encounter with highway law enforcement occurred when I was a senior in high school. I had just broken up with my steady girlfriend who lived twenty-five miles away and I was taking out my frustration on the Mississippi highway system. I was driving over seventy in a fifty-mile-per-hour zone when I was stopped. I drove the rest of the way home at a sedate fifty while clutching the evil citation in my hand. I had to report to traffic court. No mail-in fine would do.

I mulled over my problem the next day at school. Telling my parents was not an option. I would be grounded for approximately forever if they knew. Money for a fine was not a problem. I had worked before school and on weekends since seventh grade, and had always deposited part of my pay in my own bank account. I could draw out enough for my fine. All I needed was transportation to the county seat. And that was a big problem. There was no way I could use the family car. Mama's persistent, pointed questions would have wormed the truth out of me.

My deliverance appeared in the form of Gencie, a classmate, who had just turned sixteen and had access to the family car for use in our town only. I persuaded Gencie to drive me to traffic court nine miles away the next day after school. I paid my fine and listened to a lecture on highway safety, and Gencie and I returned home with neither family any wiser about our activity.

Our school annuals came out the next week, and of course everyone signed friends' books. I signed Gencie's this way: "I won't tell if you won't tell." That comment still raises eyebrows for her children and grandchildren, but Gencie has never told.

Another blue-light encounter occurred the week before my marriage. I was driving my parents and great-aunt and -uncle home from a restaurant when the blue lights flashed. I apologized for easing through the traffic light when it was a bit pink and explained to the patrolman that I was distracted because I was to be married in two days.

He said, "You have enough trouble without this ticket. I'll just give you a warning this time."

My last ticket worth mentioning occurred when I was on the faculty at Vanderbilt. I was stopped on Tyne Boulevard one afternoon as I was on my way home. I said to the policeman, "I'm so sorry I was speeding. I'm tired from a long day and besides, I was only going forty in this thirty-five-mile-per-hour zone."

The policeman replied, "I stopped you because you did a rolling stop at that four-way stop back there—but I'll just add speeding to the ticket, too."

And he did.

Some Assembly Required

Carolyn has a small office off of our upstairs den. Recently, she decided to update it. Out went the thirty year-old portable typewriter. Its only use in the last ten years has been as a toy for the grandchildren.

She needed more space for files. Only a small file cabinet could fit into the limited space available. I checked Office Depot, WalMart, Kmart, and nothing fit. All were too tall or too deep.

Carolyn searched her stack of catalogs and found just the very thing. It was small, had two drawers, was the same height as her desk, and was cheap. We ordered it that day.

About a week later, UPS delivered a long, flat box to our front porch—the file cabinet. The box measured about thirty-by-twenty-by-seven inches—not exactly a file cabinet shape. The catalog had stated, "Some assembly required." From the shape of the box, I suspected more than "some" assembly was required. Unfortunately, my suspicions were confirmed.

The box contained seventeen structural pieces and one-hundred-and-ten fasteners of twelve different types. Not one thing was attached to another. Included were three pages of assembly instructions. I was confident I could make short work of the assembly. After all, I had the instructions and had built simple furniture from raw lumber and plywood for years.

I looked at the first page of instructions.

Page one: "How to separate the glides: You should undraw the V and T, you will find a black plastic at the end. You should hold the plastic and drive up it, then undraw outside, you will find glides had been separated. Following the instruction, you will found the production is assembled easily."

I looked on the box. Yep. Made in China.

Page two: Assemble the drawer: Insert the dowel (W) into the hole of the drawer back panel (I) and Drawer side panel (F, G) rotate screw (R) into the hole of the drawer back panel (I) itset the Drawer base panel (K) follow into the Drawer side panel (FG) …

The instructions continued in this manner for a half-page. Rotating screws, haphazard punctuation, and unneeded capitalization continued unabated.

Fortunately, there was an exploded diagram, which, though difficult to fathom, was far, far easier to understand than the text.

I ignored the text and concentrated on the diagram. I made slow progress—two steps forward, one step back. It took over an hour to assemble the first drawer.

The second drawer was easier because of my experience assembling the first one. It was three steps forward and only one step back.

Then came the cabinet. Again, two steps forward, one step back. Another frustrating hour or more and "some assembly required" was done—I thought.

When I inserted the first drawer, I missed the drawer guide on one side. When I tried to withdraw the drawer, the plastic catch on the properly installed side stopped the drawer. Ah, I thought, I only have to "drive up" the plastic clip and the drawer should come out. Alas, the drawer did not open far enough to expose the clip. The drawer refused to budge despite all my efforts, forceful though they became.

Finally, I inserted a thin screwdriver in the drawer slide, lifted (drove up?) the plastic clip, and relieved the cabinet of its drawer. I carefully inserted both drawers, and the job was complete.

"Some assembly required" took all afternoon. I think the catalog writer and instruction writer should be told, "Undraw current English usage and drive up your vocabulary to found the production of better syntax."

Lamb Breast and Paper Napkins

Life is often full of surprises. Sometimes what we get is not what we think we saw.

Walking aggravate Carolyn's back problem, so I have done most of the grocery shopping the last several years. At first, I paid more attention to what was on my list than I did what each item cost. I thought a penny saved too little to worry over, especially if there might be a tax on it.

But after several years, I have become an eagle-eyed bargain seeker and glom onto bargains with the zeal of a lion after her prey. Yesterday, I even went to the customer service counter for a raincheck for a discounted item missing from the shelf. I felt a fleeting glow of consumer power as I pocketed my raincheck.

I also bought a super-large package of paper napkins for a ridiculously low price. At suppertime, I opened the package to use the napkins with our meal. We were having fried chicken, so I gave Carolyn and myself each two napkins.

Two napkins were far, far too few. At first wipe, those napkins dissolved like facial tissue. Two napkins were good for two wipes at best, wiping away any savings my smart shopping had produced.

Carolyn looked at me and said, "These napkins remind me of the lamb breast."

Back when our children were very young and I was in the military, we had shopping privileges at the Army commissary. When our youngest was newly born and Carolyn was not yet back to her usual energy level, I did the grocery shopping. After loading my cart with a month's worth of food, I stumbled upon a display of "lamb breast" at the meat counter. It was priced at five cents a pound. Who could go wrong at five cents a pound? I bought a quarter's worth.

I barbecued the ribs all Saturday afternoon, dousing them liberally with sauce. Once cooking, they emitted an aroma fit to make every mouth in the neighborhood salivate. Late that afternoon, I placed portions of the brown, sizzling ribs on our plates and we sat down to a wonderful meal of barbecued lamb.

I cut into one, then another, and another, and then, every one. There was absolutely no meat—only bone and fat and charred barbecue sauce.

Like beauty, bargains sometimes exist only in the eye of the beholder.

Packaging

We always try to make a good first impression. That's what we are told to do from our earliest adolescence. Packaging does just that in retail commerce. But things don't always turn out the way they look at first impression.

I eat quite a lot of low-calorie, low-fat, frozen entrees. I buy several whenever they are on reduced prices. They make good lunches—easy to prepare, tasty (more or less), and easy to clean up.

The packages are inviting. They display sharply focused plates of chicken or beef with broccoli, carrots, peppers, water chestnuts, and always rice or pasta. Occasionally I buy one with shrimp or salmon.

Rice and pasta abound—much more on the plate than on the package. Meat dominates the package, but is hard to find on the plate. There is spaghetti with meat sauce in the grocery freezer. Its package features a huge serving of pasta covered with a generous serving of ground beef in a thick marinara sauce. I find lots of spaghetti, little sauce. When I eat that dish I add a generous dollop of the marinara sauce I bought at Publix on special for a dime.

Today, I ate a new product. It featured shrimp and chicken in a Cajun sauce. The picture on the box was inviting—lots of thirty-count shrimp, lots of chunks of chicken, and a scattering of celery, broccoli, and peppers on a bed of rice covered with a tomato-based sauce. What a lunch. What a treat. What a disappointment.

There were a few tiny shrimp, an occasional cube of chicken, and lots of rice in a tasteless tomato sauce. I grew up close to Cajun country. This dish in no way was Cajun—not even close. Not close enough to defend the company against a lawsuit for false advertisement.

It seems I never learn. The packages continue to entice; the contents continue to disappoint; I continue to buy.

But they are convenient.

Spelling

English is such a weird language. Not only is the grammar difficult, but its spelling is impossible. It has silent letters, both at the beginnings of words and at their ends. It has double letters and fake Fs (o-u-g-h, p-h). I can spell German words and Swedish words. I can spell achromioclavicular, achrocyanosis, obliterative bronchiolitis, and monoclonal gammopathy without breaking a sweat. But, is it d-e-s-e-r-t, or is it d-e-s-s-e-r-t? D-i-n-e-r, or d-i-n-n-e-r? I often wonder. I try to avoid them. I just write, "He rode a camel through the dry, hot sandy land, toward the oasis. A piece of pie was a great way to finish my supper at the local café."

Why do we spell ladle and axle "l-e" and easel "e-l"? They sound alike but do not look alike. Why is that?

Double letters and e-l, l-e, e-r, and r-e are bad enough, but words that are spelled differently, mean different things, but sound alike make no sense to me at all. (Is it s-e-n-s-e, or c-e-n-t-s or maybe s-c-e-n-t-s? It is so confusing.)

If we shaved a grizzly, would he be a bare bear? I can't bear to see a bare bear. How about you? (Why is monkey spelled with an "e" and grizzly is not?) Would a pompous hog not be a boring boar? We could give foreign aid in lemonade, and a state department aide could distribute it.

We must wait for the proper weight of fruit to be picked. To write right, we must be a wordwright.

Our well digger will dig the whole hole even though he feels weak this week. He and his friend rode his truck down the road to the mall where they bought a new maul. They're going there in their new truck. Once out of the mall, they will meet a butcher so that he can mete out their meat. They would get some wood there, too, if he had any.

Woe is me if my horses refuse to whoa. Did you know that my team teems with great horses? I read last night until my eyes became red, but I will read again tonight.

And finally—I propped the mortgage papers against my desk so that the lien might lean a little.

An Open Letter to Mr. Cal Turner

Dear Mr. Turner,

I am writing you to ask that you consider rebuilding your barn on Franklin Road in Brentwood. I know it was unused for years and had begun to deteriorate simply from the ravages of time. But I miss it.

I have lived in Brentwood for thirty-seven years and glanced at it every time I rode down Franklin Road. It reminded me of the barn on the farm of my childhood. It, too, was green. It, too, was used primarily to store hay. I remember the oppressive heat of that enormous hayloft. Now, too, it is gone, a victim of indifferent maintenance by a series of renters. Your barn is marked by a silo, standing like a rotund headstone marking a grave. Mine disappeared into an adjacent soybean field.

Your barn has been immortalized by a photograph in the Smithsonian Institute taken by Brentwood resident Matthew Drumright. It showed a huge oil painting of a Nativity scene by Chris Tibbott. The scene covered the entire north half of the barn roof. I know you considered the barn to be your Christmas card to the citizens of Brentwood for almost twenty years. That was a fitting use for the old barn, even if some Grinch-like practical-minded citizens might deride it as a waste of money.

We in our family have a different feeling about that old relic. Some twelve years ago when my daughter, her husband, and their four children were here for their usual Christmas visit your barn was given a new name.

On Christmas Eve night, Chandler, our then three-and-a-half-year-old granddaughter looked out as we drove past the Nativity scene on the barn. She remarked, "That must be where Mary lives." From then on, whenever we passed the barn, my family thought of it, not as a barn, not as a huge Christmas card but always as "where Mary lives."

Mr. Turner, you may think it was a Christmas card, but to me and my family it will always be where Mary lives.

Mary needs a new barn.

Ten Months Later…
A Second Open Letter to Cal Turner

Dear Mr. Turner,

Thank you for rebuilding your barn in the pasture along Franklin Road. The oil painting on the barn roof every Christmas was special to all residents of Brentwood, and I know you considered the building as your Christmas card to our city. It has been immortalized in countless Christmas cards.

I watched the barn progress from partially destroyed decaying old structure to a bare spot in the pasture to the scene of resurrection. It is not a copy. It is an altogether new design and construction. It is built with Brentwood codes in mind to survive flooding of the Little Harpeth River nearby, and built to survive the worst weather short of a tornado.

I have watched the progress from a concrete slab to a series of sturdy concrete-wooden posts fastened to thick rafters with heavy custom-made brackets. It is now covered with green metal roofing. It should last approximately forever.

The old barn held a special place in the hearts of my family. Some fourteen years ago at Christmas time our then three-and-a-half-year-old granddaughter casually named the original barn. As we drove down Franklin Road on Christmas Eve she looked out at the barn covered with the Nativity scene and stated, "That's where Mary lives."

And "where Mary lives" has remained its title since. My family is overjoyed to see that Mary has a new home.

Thank you, Cal Turner.

The Morning Paper

The morning paper (the one actually printed on paper) is a rich source of ideas for this column. An issue last week was a bonanza. Here are some items I gleaned from the paper during breakfast time.

Our congresswoman, Marsha Blackburn, is without a doubt an astute politician. She seems always to say the right words, to meet with the right people, to project herself in the most effective light. She has made quite an impact on local and national politics in an incredibly short time. An example of her political acumen was covered: What better time to attack the EPA for its efforts to prevent global warming than wintertime in the midst of a major snowstorm?

The story of the two sisters serving long penal sentences in Mississippi sharing a kidney has been told earlier. Both sentences have been suspended on the condition that one sister donate a kidney to her sibling who has an end-stage renal disease. According to the paper, they are en route to Florida where their family resides. I wonder what the justice system might do if the transplanted kidney fails. Will both sisters go back to prison? Or just the donor? Or maybe the recipient? Let us hope that the question won't need to be answered.

The paper also reported that the author of the seminal study linking measles vaccine to autism has been discovered to have published fraudulent data. At least fifteen similar studies by various authors have failed to reveal any connection between vaccines and autism.

However, a vocal minority disregards those newer studies and continues to question the safety of the vaccine. Their attitude reminds me of my mother. No matter how I tried to debunk some of her pet medical pronouncements, she refused to be convinced. Her major defense was, "I don't care. I know I'm right."

And then there are the bird kill stories…

The Great American Smoke-Out

Well… you missed it. It was November nineteenth, the Great American Smoke-Out. I missed it, too. I quit for the last time, about this time of year, seventeen years ago. I had help. They stole my pants, starved me all day, and then attacked my sternum with a chainsaw. That got my attention.

I saw a cardiologist because of typical angina, and x-rays showed almost complete blockage of the main coronary artery. Complete blockage would have made my wife a widow. Emergency surgery cured me of my blockage and of my nicotine addiction. My post-op course was uneventful, though the nurses hardly thought so when I wandered off the post-op floor and set off my cardiac arrest alarm. Nobody told me my telemetry signal did not function off that floor.

After five days of a noisy room, a hard mattress, and coffee and ice cream arriving in my room at the same temperature, I came home. I was happy to be home. The nurses were happy to see me leave.

In post-op cardiac rehab, I learned that after ten years of not smoking, my life expectancy would increase to that of a lifelong non-smoker. That was something to shoot for. Now, after seventeen years without a cigarette, I have read newer and presumably more accurate statistics: those who quit after age fifty can expect to live five years longer than if they had continued to smoke. Their death rate is about half of those who continue to smoke. Not back to the risk of non-smokers, but certainly better than smokers.

I had planned to resume smoking at sixty-five, but at seventy-six I think I will leave off the cigarettes a while longer.

I plan to die from a skydiving accident at age ninety-three.

Chickens

Last month I read a newspaper article about chickens as pets. A resident of an upscale area of Davidson County had six laying hens she treated as pets. I don't see how a chicken can be a pet. I think of pets as companions who respond to their owners with affection. (Even cats will purr once in a while.) Chickens respond to an owner with disdain or fear—unless there is chicken feed in the owner's hand.

I had pets for most of my life. I have had dogs, both mutts and purebred ones. There were a rat terrier, a beagle, a sheltie, two border collies, and two mutts named Moses. The second Moses was our genius dog. More about him in another column or two.

I have also had cats—a calico who delivered kittens on Mother's Day and was an accomplished hunter. We usually ended up with a neatly dissected mouse or bird lying on our doorstep. I also had one of the dumbest cats in existence. But I digress.

I know chickens. I grew up not quite on a farm, but close enough to one for us to have a vegetable garden, a cow, and chickens—chickens for eating and chickens for eggs. I was our family's Chicken George. No, I didn't raise fighting cocks, though one of my friend's fathers did exactly that. I cared for about fifty chickens for frying, and about twenty hens for eggs. I hated every minute in the chicken pens. Pets? No way! Unpleasant chores? You bet.

The hens were for eggs. Today they would be called "free range chickens". That is, allowed to wander about a half-acre pen and scratch for seeds and insects too small to be seen by a human eye.

I gathered eggs from nesting boxes in the hen house every morning. Once or twice a year, I cleaned out the droppings from the floor beneath the roosting area. We spread the droppings on the nearby vegetable garden. Daddy swore that chicken droppings were the best garden fertilizer there was. I just swore (under my breath).

Fryers were different. We ordered just-hatched chicks from Sears every year. They arrived at our post office crowded into flat boxes. You could hear the peep-peep-peeping throughout the entire post office when they arrived.

I raised them to fryer-size in large, flat brooders. I emptied the droppings from beneath the brooders once a week. Once again, they went into the garden.

When the chickens were big enough, Mama and Grandma killed and dressed and froze all fifty of the birds. That was one day I was glad to be in school.

Hens weren't so bad. Fryers were terrible. But I ate lots of eggs and lots of fried chicken, and liked every bit of it.

Good luck with your hens, Chicken Lady. Fight the uncaring bureaucracy. Don't name your hens if you ever might want to have roast chicken.

I hope you have a garden.

Guns

Guns seem to define the Southern male's psyche. They comfort even the timid among us just knowing that stashed away in some handy (or not so handy) place lies a metallic equalizer.

We don't have a gun in our house—never had one. I doubt we ever will have one. I grew up in a non-hunting household, and so I was never infected with gun fever.

We did have a pistol in our house during my childhood. It was the result of a potential home invasion. We never locked doors at night, even though we lived next to a major highway. One night, my parents were awakened by someone opening the outside door to their bedroom. My father jumped, up grabbed a one-quart empty milk bottle from beside the door, and swatted the intruder on his head. The intruder turned and ran away. He was soon captured and proved to be a lost, drunken reveler. The very next day, my great-uncle gave my father a pistol.

The pistol languished on the top shelf in the bathroom throughout my childhood. It lay wrapped in an old towel and could be accessed only by standing on a chair. My brother-in-law retrieved it after my father died. The gun was unloaded. The grip was cracked; there were spots of rust on the barrel which was worn thin along one side of the muzzle. The barrel looked a tiny bit crooked. He felt certain the pistol would explode if fired, rendering more damage to the shooter than to the intended target. He disposed of the gun the next day.

My brother-in-law took me out one day for a pistol-shooting lesson. We shot his pistol at bottles and cans found along the bayou banks. My closest shot hit about three feet from the intended target, and the bottles and cans were anything but threatening. It seemed that the safest place for an intended victim would be directly in front of a pistol in my hands.

If I ever feel the need a gun for home protection, I would buy a short barrel pump action shotgun. It would not require careful aiming and would make a wide pattern. If I were threatened by an intruder, I would aim at his crotch. A shot there would not likely be lethal, but it would certainly get his attention.

Walking

There was an article in the newspaper some time ago analyzing walking patterns in older people. Experts explain that "trouble walking is often a sign of worse things to come." A recent study published in a medical journal stated that the slowest elderly walkers were three times more likely than their faster peers to die of heart disease within five years. I suppose walking slowly allows such infirmities to catch up with them easier.

The article goes on to state that doctors increasingly see impaired walking itself as a disorder. The National Institute on Aging in Great Britain has been given two-hundred-and-ninety-five million dollars to find out.

How about that! Walking is a disorder! And millions have been given to study this "disorder." Walking is such a natural thing that I have trouble thinking of it as a disorder. Some walk slower than others, I would admit, but almost all of us do it at one time or another.

I remember my course in physical diagnosis in medical school over fifty years ago. We even had walking mentioned in a lecture. Our teacher mentioned in passing how no longer would we notice the gait of well-put-together young women purely as a pleasurable diversion. We would forever look for disturbances in gait symptomatic of underlying illnesses. And I still do—at least, that is what I tell my wife.

The causes of many gait disturbances are easily diagnosed, at least when disturbance is pronounced. Conditions such as congenital dislocated hips, Parkinson's disease, cerebral palsy, and others betray their causes easily. Other subtle changes can be difficult to diagnose.

But walking itself as a disease? The article says that impaired walking may be a disorder itself. It seems to me that it is more likely that the walking impairment is the result of some ailment and not the cause of the problem.

The director of the institute wonders if the "disorder" is treatable, and wonders if his program "can pull them back from the brink." I wonder if there is a brink to pull them back from. But if he can pull in two-hundred-and-ninety-five million dollars, maybe there is something to this walking disease after all.

Baby Boomers

There was an article in the paper this week featuring the advent of the Baby Boomer era. According to the paper, the first baby boomers were born in January 1946, offspring of the returning service men of World War II. With their sixty-fifth birthday, they officially become old. According to today's paper, these boomers have progressed (regressed?) from senior to old. I don't know the definition of old, but maybe it's sixty-five. At least the paper says so.

To the newly old: welcome. Old isn't so bad. In fact, it's not bad at, all except body parts begin to wear out and replacements are hard to come by.

There are plusses to being old. I do not commute or make hard decisions about how to deal with difficult problems in my practice anymore. I do not set the alarm or wear a tie except on Sundays. People offer to open doors for me. (I let them.) Grocery store baggers offer to help me load my groceries. (I let them.) My children offer to drive Carolyn and me to out-of-town functions. (I let them.)

Last year, old rose up and struck me squarely in the face. My grandson asked me for a loan to help him buy an engagement ring.

My grandson was my first grandchild. Being a grandfather was a sign of impending old. Surely, I was not old enough to be a grandfather—but I was. The next seven grandchildren were easier to accept. After all, old had already entered my life.

And now, I may be a great-grandfather sometime in the future.

Being old may not be so bad after all.

Oh, What a Relief It Is

Three blissful days. Not a political ad in sight. No more pontification from reporters and commentators about this race or that one for two days. (They had to have their last licks on Wednesday to explain their errors of the previous weeks.)

Attack ads have gone into the great cyber dumpster. It feels so good not to hear words like stimulus, deficit, national debt, and jobs.

Promises flew like autumn leaves in a windstorm—and became just as hard to pin down. It seems everyone has a solution for every problem. They promise to increase jobs, decrease taxes, decrease spending, and increase services while accusing their opponent of solutions likely to lead us down the garden path to gloom and doom.

Candidates seem to promise nirvana, while their families smile self-consciously in the background as almost perceptible halos float above their heads. To hear an opponent's ads it seems we had not a single honest, hardworking, down-to-earth candidate among the lot of them.

How refreshing it would be if someone were to stroll out to a podium and modestly admit he does not have all the answers but will work hard and consult with others to arrive at possible solutions. He wishes he could perform miracles but knows he cannot. Of course, this person would be sure to lose… and big.

Now that the counting is over, the winners and losers can lean back, relax, and take stock of just what happened.

Winners will have to devise ways to squirm out of commitments made in the haste of battle, and losers will return to the task of raising money to pay for all those ads they ran on credit.

We viewers can sit back and give a sigh of relief at the absence of attack ads—at least for two years.

I'm even looking forward to the resumption of ads for cars, personal injury lawyers, pain relievers, laxatives, and remedies for erectile dysfunction.

I am Bill Fleet, and I approve this message.

Vicissitudes of Air Travel

If you haven't had problems with air transportation in your life, you haven't yet gone by air. Everyone I know has a story. Here is one of mine from my much younger days.

Early in my medical career, I spent two years doing research at the National Institutes of Health in Bethesda, Maryland. During my tenure, I wrote a research paper that was accepted for presentation at a regional virology meeting in New Orleans.

It occurred to me that I could stop by my parent's home for a short visit on my way back to Washington, and I changed my return ticket to include a stop in Greenwood, Mississippi, on Southern Air, a small regional airline not affiliated with Southwest Airlines. They landed in Greenwood, as well as other small airports.

All went well with my presentation, though I experienced near-paralysis from fear at speaking to a room full of high powered researchers. The next day, I began my odyssey on Southern Air. I think its motto should have been, "If you have time to spare fly Southern Air."

I boarded a resurrected twin engine DC-3. Even though I knew the last of these planes was built over twenty-five years before I felt not one twinge of worry. Air travel is air travel. This old plane should be as safe as any.

A half-hour flight brought us to our first stop, Biloxi, Mississippi. Landing was routine, but take-off was not. The left engine refused to start. After several minutes delay, we few passengers were asked to leave the plane. After a half-hour wait in the tiny terminal we heard an announcement, "There will be a short delay in takeoff. We can't start the port engine. Our mechanic is working on it and should have the problem fixed shortly."

"Shortly" stretched over an hour when the announcement came: "We still can't start the engine and have requested our home terminal in Atlanta to fly down our other plane." The word "other" sounded ominous. And it was.

Another announcement: "We can't start our other plane either. Our mechanic is still working on the plane here."

After about four hours, the engine started, we boarded, and we went on our way—though a few of us began to wonder where they stowed the parachutes.

After two more intermediate stops where the port engine was never shut off, we landed in Greenwood over four hours late.

My dad asked, "Why didn't they shut the left engine down when the passengers left the plane?"

He shouldn't have asked.

When my visit was over, he drove me one-hundred-and-fifty miles to Memphis to fly on a real airline back to Washington.

Red Hats, A Senior Field Trip

Last month, I became a cultured person in a half-day. I saw the current exhibition at the Frist Center for Fine Arts.

I heard of the field trip from the Martin Center by way of a casual announcement before a lecture. The announcement stated, "Get your reservations in today. Only a few places are left for the trip to the Frist Center for a guided tour." Later that day, I phoned the Martin Center to secure a reservation for Carolyn and myself, but nobody seemed to know just what I was alluding to. This response was distinctly different from the usual Martin efficiency. A few days later, I learned the date and time for the trip. We would carpool from the Martin to the Senior Center in Franklin, board a bus for the Frist Center, eat lunch there, and tour the exhibit.

We arrived at the Martin Center a bit early with our friend Joyce, picked up passengers, including Virginia, a writer-friend, and headed toward Franklin. At the Franklin center, we walked into a room filled by over thirty gray-haired, purple-clad, red-hatted women, all wearing sensible shoes and chatting and laughing like schoolgirls. We had joined, unknowingly, the Red Hat Society. They had organized the trip and needed a few Martin Center members to fill their bus. I was the lone male. Now I know what it feels like to be in a minority.

Lunch was without incident, but I noticed that chatter diminished significantly. Entering the exhibit hall was an altogether different matter. Our docent found it difficult to believe I was a Red Hat (however pro tem), and asked me to leave the group. Only after the chief Red Hat vouched for me was I allowed to participate.

Our docent was so very well-versed on the exhibit that I asked her at the tour's conclusion if she had studied art or art appreciation in college.

"No," she replied, "I am a lawyer."

Who would have thought it?

On the bus ride home, I listened to plans for the next outing, a trip to Tunica. Where can I find a purple vest and a red hat?

Not a Hero—Not

My friend's book begins this way: "How in the hell did I get into this mess—plane's all shot up, tires are flat, no brakes, wounded crew trying to survive… and, thirty of our planes behind us are depending on me to lead them back to our base! Even if we do make it back, how am I going to land this sucker?"

My friend, a fellow Brentwood resident, had a birthday last month. It was his ninetieth. I looked in the Tennessean for a mention of his birthday. There was none. The paper seems mostly to include show business people and seldom mentions heroes. My friend was a hero. It's a shame his memoir is out of print.

Jim was born in Canada and became a naturalized U.S. citizen at age 20. Pearl Harbor was bombed when he was twenty-one. He was called into the Army at twenty-two. He insists he applied for the Air Corps only because he preferred a warm bed and warm food over mud and cold rations.

He passed flight training without difficulty and qualified for fighter aircraft. However, because of the needs of the Army he was assigned to fly bombers. He always equated bombers as clumsy bomb haulers, and when asked what he did in the war, he usually replied that he was a truck driver. He delivered bombs.

If he was a truck driver, he was a good one. He completed twenty-five missions piloting B24s—a lumbering four engine bomber that was much more difficult to fly and had a less romantic image than the B17, the "Flying Fortress." He never lost a plane or a crewman.

Jim showed such outstanding leadership qualities during bombing missions that he became a leader of his squadron of twelve planes after only a few missions. He flew most of his later missions as a leader of groups of bombers up to one-hundred-and-forty-four planes. Toward the end of his tour, he and his crew only flew as leader of his division which consisted of five-hundred planes when at peak strength.

He flew as leader of his group of thirty-two planes on the famous Gotha raid deep inside Germany. His leadership resulted in a highly successful raid where ninety percent of the target, the Messerschmitt Aircraft works was destroyed or heavily damaged. His unit received a presidential unit citation for the raid.

Ask Jim if he was a hero and he denies it. Ask him if he won any medals and he replies, "I had a few but I don't remember what they were."

I will tell you what they were:

Presidential Unit Citation

Distinguished Flying Cross, (four times). This medal is the highest medal short of the Medal of Honor given for acts performed while in flight.

Air Medal, (five times)

He claims that he is no hero, that he had a job to do, and he did it as best he could.

I disagree. He was a hero who did his job heroically.

Huff's

I was saddened to read of Mr. Glen Huff's recent death. I read tributes to the man and his wife in both the Brentwood Homepage and the Tennessean. Both papers were lavish in their praise of both him this family, and it was richly deserved. However, I read only a little about Huff's (the grocery).

The grocery was in the Huff family for many, many years until Mr. Huff retired in 1987 and his son Mike sold the store building in 1993 to the business currently occupying it. This building was roomy, attractive, and inviting. But it was not the Huff's I had grown to love.

The older Huff's occupied the nearby building that houses Inside/Outside today. I became acquainted with Huff's shortly after my family and I moved to Brentwood in 1974. I recall my first visit to the store. It held much of the charm and ambience of a country grocery of an even earlier time. It was small for a supermarket and needed better lighting. Space was severely limited and aisles needed signs announcing one-way traffic. If you met another customer, one of you had to back out to an intersection to allow the other customer to continue shopping. The building had been enlarged more than once, and floors sloped between newer and older sections. A shopper turned his back on his cart at his peril. Often the uninitiated failed to maintain a hold on his cart, and when the new patron looked back he found his cart trundling down the sloping aisle.

Mr. Huff and his number one associate, Frank, wore long white aprons reminiscent of earlier days before World War II. I don't recall ever seeing one wear a dirty apron, even behind the meat counter. Young employees carried your groceries to your car without being asked.

Huff's was unique in many ways, but it was the only grocery outside of my hometown country store that functioned somewhat like our local bank. It maintained charge accounts for regular customers and allowed children to charge items to their parent's accounts as well. (Of course, Mr. Huff and Frank knew every adult and child in the small town of Brentwood.)

Banks were closed at night and on weekends, and ATMs had not been invented yet when we moved here. However, being caught short of cash was never a problem. Mr. Huff or Frank gladly advanced a twenty-dollar-bill or two on request of good customers. They merely added the cash advance to our monthly tab.

When Huff's moved, I always felt a bit uneasy. Even though Mr. Huff and Frank and Mike were there, the new store felt strange. It just wasn't the same without cramped aisles and runaway carts. I even was reluctant to ask for credit.

Apocalyptic Talk

Last month we endured unending talk about end times—the time when the earth and all in it would be destroyed and only a small number of us would qualify for inclusion in the new world.

The principal author of this discussion was a Bible scholar on the West Coast who had it all figured out. He predicted with great assurance that the world as we know it would end on a certain day in the late spring of 2011. Some people sold or gave away all their worldly possessions and stood ready to go. The Bible scholar missed his date (proven by my writing about it today and by you reading—if you have gotten this far.)

After the fateful date passed, the Bible scholar announced he had miscalculated and it would be in October this year, 2012. I guess the faithful breathed a sigh of relief for the reprieve. I expect the super-faithful had regrets about the loss of their property—but maybe not. After all, they would be gone in only a few months later than they had hoped.

I have been a practicing Christian for over sixty years, in a mainstream denomination, and have never been worried about the end times. I take comfort in New Testament statements that nobody knows when the end times will come.

In the week before the supposed end time, I saw a bumper sticker on a pickup truck parked in the patient's parking garage near a multi-story medical office building. The sticker said, "When the rapture comes, this vehicle will be empty." I wondered that, if the end times were so near, why bother to go to the doctor?

I have wondered this about the rapture for some time: What if the rapture really came, and nobody qualified? Who would know?

A final thought: If the world does not come to an end in October as is predicted, and if the lockout wipes out the NFL season, a few rabid Titan fans may think the world has indeed come to the end, anyway.

Limbo

Today I helped in a small way with the memorial service for an extremely premature baby who died on his third day of life. The service brought back memories of similar sad days in my own pediatric practice.

During my first week of residency at the Philadelphia Children's Hospital, I was told that, when a baby died, to baptize him with sterile water taken from a previously unopened bottle. This sort of baptism is considered valid, even in the eyes of the Roman Catholic Church. It did not require ordained clergy or Holy Water or even a communicant in the Catholic Church. From then on, throughout my pediatric career, I did just that, though I never questioned why it was so important.

Recently, I ran across an article in the New York Times that explained why infant baptism is so important in the eyes of the Catholic Church. To the Church, unbaptized babies are consigned to Limbo, a place outside Heaven. Unlike Purgatory, Limbo is not a temporary way station for people who eventually reach Heaven. Limbo is a permanent blissful state outside Heaven, close to God but not in communion with God.

Though the concept of Limbo has no basis in Scripture, it has remained a part of Catholic Church for over fifteen-hundred years. Recently, the concept of Limbo has been challenged once again, but still it holds sway.

While belief in God may not change, the things people believe about God certainly do. As a concept, Limbo has long been relegated to a minor status, an interesting relic. But now it has reemerged in importance. The Catholic Church is growing fastest among the poor of Africa and Asia, where spontaneous abortion rates and infant death rates remain high. Priests can console mothers by explaining that fetuses and newborn babies who lose their lives unbaptized will experience eternity, if not with God, at least close to God. Anything that comforts people who have lost their babies cannot be too bad.

I am not Roman Catholic. But still, even in overwhelmingly Protestant Middle Tennessee, every time I presided over the death of a young baby, I always baptized the little soul.

I always told the parents what I had done. Seldom did the knowledge of the baptism comfort them. Limbo rarely entered into parents' thinking. But still, it always made me feel better to do it. I had done everything I could for the baby during life, and even after life.

I could cure sometimes. I could comfort sometimes. I could do my best to do both, always.

Full Circle

My wife and I are church mice. Church mice are never seen. You only know they have been there by what they leave behind. We prepare the sanctuary for Sunday worship services once a month.

Last month, we arrived just as the funeral of a Brentwood college student had ended. We entered the sanctuary feeling as though we were interlopers or voyeurs. Dozens of damp tissues littered the pews and the floor in the area where family and close friends had been sitting. As we cleaned, we picked up warm tears of grief and love and briefly held them in our hands.

We replaced the altar cloth and the pulpit cloth and carefully folded the simple pall. It is very plain and is used in every funeral here to signify that we are all equal before God. We moved the Pascal candle from the center of the chancel-rail to its usual place beside the baptismal font. It is lit only at funerals, baptisms, and on Easter morning and Christmas Eve.

Next, feeling rather subdued, we tackled the pews. As we straightened hymnals and replaced prayer-request cards, envelopes and other supplies, our minister of music entered from a side door accompanied by a beaming young couple. Before we had finished, we heard excerpts of traditional wedding music and a happy dialogue as the couple selected the music for their wedding.

"There is a time to be born and a time to die,
A time to plant and a time to uproot.
A time to weep and a time to laugh,
A time to mourn and a time to dance."
(Ecclesiastes, Chapter 3)

The Day the Lights Went Out in Brentwood

There I was, sitting at the breakfast table in my pajamas, just as calm as you please. I had just about finished my second cup of coffee when a loud boom reverberated through the house and all our lights went out.

What happened? Was it a car wreck, or maybe a bomb? It was surely loud enough for a bomb. Maybe a terrorist attack. Our Brentwood power grid was certainly vulnerable, and it is vital to the lives of us Brentwoodites. Terrorists had attacked New York and Washington. Why not Brentwood?

I peeped out the back door toward the direction of the boom. No smoke. No people. No flashing lights. Nothing out of the ordinary. A look out the front door revealed the same.

What's going on? Nothing seems unusual except we had no power. No power anywhere. No lights, no furnace, no stove, no refrigerator, no microwave. And… no oatmeal and no toast, my usual breakfast.

There seemed to be no obvious threat. But the crisis continued. What to fix for breakfast? And it a Sunday, and I was an usher this month. I did what most suburban heads of household do: I asked the real head of our household as she walked through the kitchen on her way to fetch our battery-powered lantern.

She said, "There're Wheaties in the pantry and milk in the refrigerator. You'll survive. I need to dress for church."

After a few crackers with peanut butter for breakfast, I staggered down the hall to our bedroom, flipping light switch after light switch without success. I reached into my closet and selected my wedding-and-funeral suit and sincere tie by feel and dressed by our ever-dimming lantern. We made it to church on time, and arrived back at home to find everything the way it should be. No sirens, no troops, no damage to any power pole that I could see. We had power enough for furnace, lights, and everything, enough for me to warm last night's dinner for lunch—and to type this column.

Random Unconnected Thoughts

The only people who know the metric system seem to be scientists and dealers in illicit drugs.

If a retired person takes a vacation, does it mean he goes back to work for two weeks?

Our country's trade deficit is becoming serious. Recently we bought some China. It was made in China.

I just became a year older; I had to add another pill.

There are no Danish Pastries in Denmark.

I have my little rebellious traits. Instead of removing credit cards from readers quickly as the instructions say, I always remove them very, very slowly.

I saw an article in the paper that stated, "Over fifty percent of the population of Texas is Latino minorities." If that is so, how can they be minorities?

I am going to have to change churches. Our church is advertising a kids sale (no apostrophe). I do not think selling children is a legitimate activity for a church.

Is there any way we can limit global warming to wintertime?

Have you ever seen a jogger whose face did not reflect misery?

Have you noticed? Everyone at the "Y" parks as close to the entrance as they can when they go for a workout.

I never knew I had so many friends until I bought a pickup truck.

Last Sunday, the referee signaled "unnecessary roughness" in a football game. Can anyone tell me just what "necessary roughness" is?

I have noticed that every deer hunter pictured in the paper is wearing camouflaged pants and shirts topped by day glow orange vests and caps—sort of a sartorial oxymoron.

It seems that everytime I am running late to an appointment, every traffic light is red. When I am early, every light seems to be green.

I just finished reading a biography of Dorothy Parker. There are two hundred pages of unforgettable quotes. I can't remember a single one of them. Who is Dorothy Parker, anyway?

Advice to do something good for myself always calls for something that is uncomfortable, expensive, or tastes bad.

Happiness Is:

I was asked to write a short essay in my writer's seminar on happiness.

Everyone chases happiness. Everyone wants some. Even the Declaration of Independence promises to promote happiness— or at least the pursuit of happiness. No guarantee; just the pursuit.

What makes you happy? Is it a warm puppy or a purring kitten in your lap? Puppies and kittens, like humans, grow and become adults. Like humans, they are sometimes difficult to live with.

We know lots of things happiness is not, and few things happiness really is. Happiness usually does not come from stuff, yet we seem ever to acquire more things. My father often said about possessions, "All I want is my land, and all the land that touches it. Of course he said it with tongue firmly planted in his cheek.

Happiness often doesn't last in marriage. If it did, why is the divorce rate about fifty percent?

Happiness sometimes doesn't come from children. Some children can be less a joy and more a trial.

So, what is this illusive thing we call happiness? I think happiness may be contentment—the feeling of satisfaction with what we have and the feeling of pleasure in how we live and in the warmth of love.

If I Were

I was asked recently to discuss who I would be if I had my life to live over. If I were not me, who would I be?

I never wanted to be a policeman or a fireman. I never saw either of those men. We didn't have them where I grew up. Our town was too small for fires or crime.

I never wanted to follow my father's calling. Surely, I wouldn't be a farmer. They work too hard in the hot sun and they get up too early. I worked part-time in my father's business, but that never appealed to me, either.

I hung around the crop duster field, and flew a time or two, and even made innumerable model airplanes, but I never considered flying as a career.

Maybe it was the local family practitioner that caught my eye. He had a ready laugh and a vast store of stories. But I don't think he was the source of my interest in medicine. I just knew medicine was for me from my earliest memories.

Not that there were other enticements. I was a decent tennis player, but I knew that recreational tennis was as far as I could go. My college freshman English teacher tried to convince me to change majors to English and become a writer, but somehow I knew writing would be another hobby at best.

And so I did the medical-school thing and ended up with a practice full of babies and children. I didn't come close to becoming rich, but I earned enough to live comfortably. I enjoyed my patients and most of their mothers. Of course, grandmothers and I usually eyed each other warily. Pediatricians and grandmothers are natural enemies. We both are experts in rearing children.

What would I be if I were someone different? Would I be some other kind of doctor? Or perhaps not a doctor at all. But what else? I don't think I could make a living as a writer. So, what would I be?

If I had it to do over again, I think I would just do it over again.

Afterword

I'm finished, done, and all used up word-wise. Carolyn asked me what will I do in my afternoons now.

I thought a moment and replied, "I guess I'll go back to making birdhouses."